MODERN
CHINESE EAR
ACUPUNCTURE

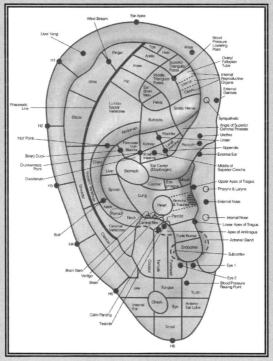

PING CHEN

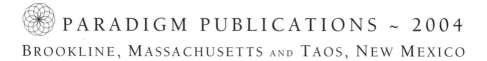

PARADIGM PUBLICATIONS ~ 2004

BROOKLINE, MASSACHUSETTS AND TAOS, NEW MEXICO

Modern Chinese Ear Acupuncture

Translated and amended by Ping Chen

Edited by Michael Helme

Copyright ©2004 Paradigm Publications

ISBN 0-912111-70-4

Library of Congress Cataloging-in-Publication Data

Chen, Ping, 1953-
  Modern Chinese ear acupuncture / Ping Chen ; [translated and amended
by Ping Chen ; edited by Michael Helme].
      p. ; cm.
Includes bibliographical references and index.
Translated from Chinese.
  ISBN 0-912111-70-4
  1. Ear--Acupuncture.
  [DNLM: 1. Acupuncture, Ear. 2. Medicine, Chinese Traditional. WB
369.5.E2 C518m 2003a] I. Helme, Michael. II. Title.
  RM184 .C48247313 2003
  615.8'92--dc21
                          2003001439

Published by Paradigm Publications
www.paradigm-pubs.com
Distributed by Redwing Book Company
202 Bendix Drive
Taos, New Mexico 87571
www.redwingbooks.com

TABLE OF CONTENTS

EDITOR'S FOREWORD

My thanks to Dr. Chen Ping for the opportunity I have had to work with her in the course of editing this text.

Because her work has always included clinical practice, she has excellent first-hand knowledge of ear both from a clinical and theoretical standpoint. When Dr. Chen began teaching Chinese medicine to English-speaking students in the U.S. (at the International Institute of Chinese Medicine in Albuquerque, New Mexico), she discovered that their ability to learn was severely curtailed by the poor quality of their texts and written materials. Sensitive to her student's needs, she was moved to translate and compose useful, reliable texts for them.

The book you have in your hands grew out of Dr. Chen's effort to improve the understanding of ear acupuncture among English readers and is thus enriched and enlivened by her experience as a doctor, translator, and teacher. Because she has dedicated so much effort and energy to her study of medicine and to making information available for our study, she deserves our full gratitude.

NATURE OF THE TRANSLATION

This text is not a direct translation. Although professional translation standards have been applied, the original manuscript has been substantively edited in preparation. In preparing this text, Dr. Chen began with a Chinese manuscript on ear acupuncture that was intended for professional clinicians who would exclusively practice ear acupuncture. Dr. Chen then selected and translated what was useful for Western clinicians and conscienciously eliminated procedures in the original text that were inapplicable in the Western environment. As a result, and because of Dr. Chen's extensive knowledge of the subject within the larger practice of Chinese medicine, *Modern Chinese Ear Acupuncture* is precisely directed to the needs and clinical circumstances of its readers.

HISTORY OF EAR ACUPUNCTURE

Chapter One of this text includes an overview of the history of ear acupuncture. That overview states what virtually every source in China says about ear acupuncture: it is a method of healing with roots that go deep into the history of China and Chinese medicine. For the sake of Western readers who are familiar with Dr. Paul Nogier's original works on auriculotherapy, as well as Dr. Terry Oleson's eclectic and comprehensive work on the international traditions of ear acupuncture and auriculotherapy, various facts and observations on the history of ear acupuncture follow.

Ear Acupuncture Versus Auriculotherapy

People often use the terms "ear acupuncture" and "auriculotherapy" as synonymous. However, if we refer to the use of ear-centered therapy in China as "ear acupuncture" and to its use in Europe, America, and other non-Asian countries as "auriculotherapy," we can clarify, compare and contrast of the history of this treatment.

The histories of auriculotherapy and ear acupuncture are closely interrelated. It is generally agreed that Dr. Paul Nogier, M.D., is the founder of auriculotherapy. Having observed several patients with ear scars from a folk-treatment that had successfully cured sciatica pain, Dr. Nogier investigated this treatment, theorized how it might work, and eventually conceived of the ear as a microsystem of the entire body that reflects illnesses of the body and allows for their treatment. Dr. Nogier acknowledges that in the course of his investigations he spoke with a Chinese person who performed such treatments. Moreover, an acupuncture-like needle is the primary auriculotherapy treatment.

Auriculotherapy, as defined here, is a form of Western alternative medicine. It uses the anatomy of Western medicine and the pathologies of Western medicine, and attempts to heal these diseases with an alternative method. The primary underlying insight of auriculotherapy, that the whole of the body could be diagnosed and treated within a single part of the whole, is an expression of a holistic ideal that has been expressed by many.

Literature from the People's Republic of China recognizes Dr. Nogier's contribution to auriculotherapy, while noting that ear acupuncture is a very ancient and traditional part of Chinese medicine. Not only the text translated for this book, but other Chinese sources, say that in 1958 the first complete auriculotherapy chart, which originated with Dr. Nogier, was published in a German journal, made its way to China, and quickly gained wide recognition. Soon after, there began a review of the

Chinese classics, and much clinical practice and study. However, the perspective in China has always been that ear acupuncture is rooted in the history of Chinese medicine.

Despite differing views on the origins of ear acupuncture, everyone accepts it is an integral part of modern clinical acupuncture practice. Moreover, part of the long tradition of Chinese medicine has been the acceptance of new therapies that work—even when the theory and concepts supporting them are different from the theories and concepts that support other successful therapies.

Michael Helme, January 2003

ABOUT THE AUTHOR

Dr. Ping Chen, a native of Anhui Province, earned a Western medical doctorate at the Shandong Medical University with a specialization in cardiology. Subsequently she received a degree in Chinese medicine with a specialty in Chinese herbal therapy from the Shandong Traditional Chinese Medicine University. Upon completion of her studies, she was made a professor at both Shandong Medical University and Shandong TCM University. In China she was widely known and highly regarded for her command of English and her skills in translating texts on Chinese medicine. From 1992 to 1998 she translated and published over one hundred books and innumerable articles on Chinese medicine to facilitate the studies of foreign students visiting China.

Dr. Chen presently treats patients and hosts seminars at the Yi Ling Medical Center, a leading medical clinic for the application of and instruction in Chinese medicine in the United States. An energetic and resourceful teacher and clinician, she is favored with respect and admiration from her students and patients.

DESIGNATION

In Council of Oriental Medical Publishers terms this text is a compilation of an original work with translation based on the *Practical Dictionary of Chinese Medicine* by Wiseman and Feng, Paradigm Publications, Brookline, Massachusetts, 1998.

CHAPTER ONE

INTRODUCTION

THE ORIGIN AND DEVELOPMENT OF EAR ACUPUNCTURE

Origin

Ear acupuncture refers to the therapeutic method of using filiform needles, vaccaria seeds, or other devices or procedures to stimulate ear points so as to reach the goal of healing. It is an important component of traditional Chinese acupuncture and moxibustion.

Ear acupuncture originated in China. Before the *Inner Cannon (Nèi Jīng)* was written, ancient practitioners of Chinese medicine had accumulated a wealth of knowledge and experience in treating diseases with ear acupuncture.

The Classic of Acupuncture and Moxibustion along Eleven Channels of the Legs and Arms (Zú Bì Shí Yī Mài Jiu Jīng) and *Classic of Acupuncture and Moxibustion along Eleven Yin and Yang Channels (Yīn Yáng Shí Yī Mài Jiu Jīng)*, the earliest known writings on acupuncture and moxibustion, were unearthed in 1973 at Han Tomb 3, Ma Wang Dui, Changsha, in the People's Republic of China. Their discussion of the use of ear points for treatments related to the upper limbs, eyes, cheeks, and throat clearly show that people of that time had an initial understanding of ear acupuncture.

In the *Inner Canon* there are 95 references to the ear. *Magic Pivot* (*Líng Shū*)[1] not only records the treatment principles of ear acupuncture, it also includes descriptions of ear points and indications for treatments by needling the ear. For example, *Magic Pivot* indicates the use of point Ear Center in treating deafness. The earliest records of ear diagnosis were also found in *Magic Pivot*, where it is recorded, "A parched and desiccated helix that looks dirty or dusky (hyperpigmentation) shows that the disease is related to bone," and "a protruding, green-blue vessel in the ear is seen in convulsion."

These references indicate there is a very long history behind ear acupuncture and that this special form of therapy must have originated in China.

Development

While ear acupuncture originated during the Spring and Autumn Period as well as the Warring States Period, later practitioners vastly broadened its application. For example, in the field of ear diagnosis, Yang Shang-Shan, a famous physician in the Sui Dynasty, wrote in *Inner Canon Great Collection* (*Huáng Dì Nèi Jīng Dà Sù*), "The front of the ear [referring to the area around Lower Apex of Tragus (MA-T2)] feels hot if the disease is related to the small intestine." He also wrote, "A patient with reverting yīn headache will feel heat in the front and posterior surface of the ear." Also Huang-Fu Mi, a famous physician in the Jing Dynasty, wrote in *Classic of Acupuncture and Moxibustion* (*Zhēn Jiŭ Jiă Yĭ Jīng*), "A protruding, green-blue vessel in an infant's ear indicates convulsions and abdominal pain, as well as diarrhea with undigested food in the stools."

Ancient practitioners of Chinese medicine also accumulated a wealth of experience in treating diseases with ear acupuncture. For example, Gĕ Hóng, another famous physician in the Jing Dynasty, wrote in *Zhŏu Hòu Bèi Jí Fāng* (*Emergency Standby Remedies*), "Bloodletting at Ear Center and Internal Nose with Chinese onion will treat cerebral bleeding and cerebral thrombosis and shock." Sun Si-Miao, a famous physician in the Tang Dynasty, wrote in *A Thousand Gold Pieces Prescriptions* (*Bèi Jí Qiān Jīn Yào Fāng*), "Ear Center can be used to treat yáng jaundice as well as cold and damp epidemic diseases . . ." Yang Ji-Zhou, a famous physician in the Ming Dynasty, wrote in *The Great Compendium of Acupuncture and Moxibustion* (*Zhēn Jiŭ Dà Chéng*): "Moxibustion at Ear Apex will treat cataracts; use

---

[1] *Magic Pivot* is the second of two parts that comprise the *Inner Cannon*.

five small cones of moxibustion." He also wrote: "Needling with a filiform needle at Ear Gate [TB-21] can treat tooth pain."

Ear acupuncture continued to develop throughout the Qing Dynasty. Zhang Di-Shan described in detail how to use the auricle to diagnose diseases in his book titled *Essential Techniques for Massage* (*Lǐ Zhèng Àn Mò Yào Shù*). The first chart of ear points can be found in this book.

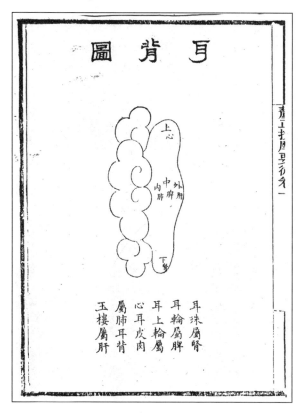

Figure 1.1: Illustration from a Qing Dynasty text by Zhang Di-Shan, *Essential Techniques for Massage* (*Lǐ Zhèng Àn Mò Yào Shù*).

Ear acupuncture has also made the following rapid advances since the founding of the People's Republic of China:

(1) With the development of medical sciences, TCM and Western medicine have begun to influence each other. In 1956 Paul Nogier, a French doctor, drew a chart of ear points that was mapped from the shape of an inverted fetus. This was the first complete ear point chart in history. The introduction of that chart to China in 1958 initiated many developments in ear acupuncture. These developments include thorough research of historical Chinese medical literature and the development of a unique

system of ear diagnosis and acupuncture treatments, with a variety of treatment procedures.

(2) Numerous theses, journals, and monographs on ear acupuncture have been published.

(3) Specialized departments have been established in schools, clinics, and hospitals to train and employ ear acupuncture specialists.

(4) In 1982, the Ear Acupuncture Division of the Chinese Acupuncture Association was established to cultivate ear acupuncture research and dissemination. In the middle of the 1980s, the *International Standardized Scheme of Ear Points* that was published in China was distributed abroad and widely accepted by the international medical community. In 1992, *Standardized Names and Location of Ear Points* was published. All these measures promoted the development and standardization of ear acupuncture.

(5) Specific diagnostic techniques related to the ear have also been developed. Apart from traditional ear inspection, advances were made in ear point palpation and electrodetection.

(6) Apart from traditional needling with filiform needles and the application of moxibustion, other variations on ear acupuncture have been developed, including seed pressing, needle implantation, and medicinal injection. More than 200 kinds of disorders have been treated with ear acupuncture, including internal, external, gynecological, obstetric, pediatric, eye, nose, ear, mouth, and skin disorders; ear acupuncture has also been used for anesthesia. In general ear acupuncture has an 85 percent effectiveness rate, and 60 different disorders can be treated with a 60 percent complete cure rate.

Clinical data shows that ear acupuncture is easy to learn, is effective, and is free of side effects. It can be used in the prevention, diagnosis, and treatment of many disorders.

Ear acupuncture is also well known internationally. In countries including France, Germany, Italy, the United Kingdom, the United States, Canada, Australia, Russia, Japan, Korea, and India, ear acupuncture has been researched and applied in treatments for several decades. Academic activities such as international conferences and training classes are becoming more and more widespread, while an increasing number of books on ear acupuncture have been published in China and in many other countries.

Theoretical Explanations of Ear Acupuncture

At present there is no clear physical explanation of how ear acupuncture works. Neural, neurochemical, biochemical, bioelectrical, and other approaches have all been researched, yet no one has presented a compelling scientific explanation or even made a significant contribution to how ear points should be selected or treated through science-based measures. According to the traditional Chinese theories of the channels and network vessels, and of the bowels and viscera, the ears (and all other parts of the body) are connected and related to all other parts of the body. In fact, some practitioners regard specific parts of the body, such as the soles of the feet, as microsystems of the entire body that can be used to treat the entire body. Yet this still begs the question of a specific mechanism explaining how ear acupuncture (or foot acupuncture) works.

In China, Professor Zhang Ying Qing is credited with establishing the theory of Embryonic Complete Information of the Holistic Organ. One aspect of this is the theory of holism, which in holistic medicine means that a living organism is correctly seen as a whole that is more than the sum of its constituent parts. Another aspect of this theory is that (1) information from embryonic representations of an organism can reveal a complete diagnostic picture, and (2) applying treatments on such an embryonic representation can supply the body with the "information" it needs to cure itself.

When studying and applying ear acupuncture it can be instructive to recall that while there is no explanation for how it works, it does work. Patients are cured of some diseases with ear acupuncture. Yet like most therapies in Chinese medicine, we must simply respect the experiences of other physicians and learn from our own successes and failures in order to make it a useful therapy for relieving illness.

CHARACTERISTICS AND INDICATIONS OF EAR ACUPUNCTURE

Characteristics of Ear Acupuncture

WIDE RANGE OF APPLICATIONS AND QUICK THERAPEUTIC EFFECT

Ear acupuncture may be used for both diagnosis and treatment of internal and external conditions, traumatic injury, and musculoskeletal, gynecological, obstetric and pediatric diseases, as well as disorders of the eye, ear, nose, and throat. In addition, it can strengthen the body's resistance to disease and prevent invasion of pathogens, promote longevity, and enhance physical beauty. It can also be used as an anesthetic. According to one study, more than 200 kinds of diseases and disorders can be treated with ear acupuncture.

EASY TO LEARN AND PRACTICE

The rules for locating ear points are easily mastered. Thus, most of the methods introduced in this book are suitable not only for experienced medical practitioners, but also for lay people who are interested in ear acupuncture.

SAFE AND FREE FROM HARMFUL SIDE EFFECTS

Ear acupuncture is one of the safest of all external therapies. It allows the patient to avoid medicines and/or invasive surgical procedures that may cause other kinds of physical damage. Ear acupuncture has almost no side effects, not even the accidental needle breakage or local needle impacting that occasionally happens during body acupuncture.

INEXPENSIVE AND CONVENIENT

Ear acupuncture is an inexpensive therapy because it requires no special medical facilities. Filiform needles, a three-edged needle, vaccaria seeds, alcohol wipes, and bandages are the only tools and materials required. Because it may be performed anywhere a patient needs medical care (even at home), costly and difficult clinical visits can therefore be avoided.

Primary Indications for Ear Acupuncture

VARIOUS PAIN DISORDERS

Traumatic disorders:
Sprains and contusions, stab wounds, cuts, fractures, joint dislocations, gangrene of fingers or toes, crick in the neck, scalds.

Inflammatory conditions
Tonsillitis, pharyngitis, mastitis, phlebitis, angitis, erysipelas, prostatitis, cystitis, rheumatoid arthritis.

Post-surgical pain
Pain occurring in openings, scars, and phantom pain.

Neuralgia
Supraorbital neuralgia, trigeminal neuralgia, migraine, intercostal neuralgia, post-therapeutic neuralgia, sciatica.

Tumor pain
Pain occurring in various kinds of cancer or tumors.

INFLAMMATORY DISEASES

Acute conjunctivitis, keratitis, electric ophthalmia, periodontitis, otitis media, laryngopharyngitis, tonsillitis, parotitis, lobar pneumonia, pleuritis, bronchitis, gastritis, enteritis, appendicitis, cholecystitis, pelvic inflammation, cervicitis, orchitis, epididymitis, peripheral neuritis.

ALLERGIES AND COLLAGEN DISEASES

Allergic rhinitis, allergic asthma, allergic purpura, irritable colitis, erythema nodosum, rheumatoid arthritis, drug rash, urticaria, lupus erythematosus.

DISORDERS CAUSED BY DISTURBANCES OF THE NERVOUS SYSTEM AND THE ENDOCRINE SYSTEM

Hysteria, neurosis, Menière's syndrome, hypertension, arrhythmia, gastrointestinal disorders, sexual disorders, climacteric syndrome, sterility, dysmenorrhea, amenorrhea, dysfunctional uterine bleeding, seminal emission, impotence, prostatitis, enuresis, hyperthyroidism, diabetes, obesity, acne, bromhidrosis, chloasma.

CHRONIC DISEASES

Chronic pain in the lumbus and legs, omalgia, cervical spondylopathy, myofibrositis, chronic persistent hepatitis, post-concussion syndromes, post-trauma brain syndromes, chronic cholecystitis, chronic gastritis, duodenal ulcer.

INFECTIOUS DISEASES

Influenza, mumps, whooping cough, scarlet fever, tuberculosis, bacterial dysentery, infectious hepatitis, epidemic encephalitis B, and pubertal flat warts.

OTHER DISEASES

Ear acupuncture can also be used for coccygeal disorders, stimulation of lactation, substance abuse withdrawal (including alcohol, tobacco, and drugs), food poisoning, and competition anxiety. It can also prevent transfusion reactions and motion sickness, as well as the common cold. It is also helpful for bodybuilding, physical beauty, and weight loss.

In general, ear acupuncture has a wide range of applications; it can heal or alleviate many diseases.

POINTS FOR ATTENTION AND CONTRAINDICATIONS

Points for Attention

- The treatment method selected should always be suitable to the patient's condition.
- Strict sterilization procedures should be followed when using filiform needles, needle implantation, point-cutting,[2] bloodletting, and other methods to avoid infections.
- Ear acupuncture should not be performed if the patient has an empty stomach, has overeaten or overstrained, or has profuse bleeding.
- Strong stimulation from forceful manipulations and invasive methods such as picking therapy[3] should be avoided in older adults and those who are particularly sensitive. Should fainting occur it should be dealt with promptly.
- People with hypertension, coronary heart disease, and arteriosclerosis should be adequately rested before ear acupuncture is applied.
- Sensitive spots should be detected before point manipulation begins, as treating sensitive spots is more effective.

Apart from these general considerations, each different treatment method has special considerations that will be introduced in the following chapters and sections.

Contraindications

Ear acupuncture is very safe and, generally speaking, there are no absolute contraindications. However, the following concerns should be recalled:

- Avoid strong stimulation for patients with severe heart disease.
- Only seed acupressure can be used for patients with severe, chronic diseases, particularly for those who tend to bleed or have severe anemia.
- Ear acupuncture should not be performed if the ear has dermal disorders.

---

[2] *Editor's note*: "Point cutting" is a therapeutic technique performed by cutting at a point and removing a little fatty tissue.

[3] *Editor's note*: "Picking therapy" is a therapeutic technique performed using a three-edged needle to break a small amount of fibrous tissue at the point or area so that a small amount of blood surfaces.

- Ear acupuncture is contraindicated for at least the first trimester of pregnancy. Following the fifth month of pregnancy, mild stimulation may be used. The points Internal Reproductive Organs (MA-TF), Abdomen (MA-AH), and Endocrine (MA-IC3) should not be treated.

COMMONLY SEEN REACTIONS TO TREATMENT AND MANAGEMENT OF ACUPUNCTURE ACCIDENTS

Commonly Seen Reactions to Treatment

Because the ear is where channels and nerves gather, treatments applied in the ear can induce a variety of treatment responses throughout the body.

TREATMENT RESPONSES IN THE EAR

Obvious pain will be felt in the ear in most cases when points are treated. Soreness, numbness, distention, and coldness may be felt in some instances. Later, congestion and heat will be felt at the treated points or even throughout the ear. These reactions are considered "obtaining qì" in ear acupuncture. In general, patients who have this kind of response have received an effective treatment.

TREATMENT RESPONSES IN THE REGION OF DISEASE

The body area or part that has disease will sometimes feel hot and/or uncomfortable when the corresponding ear points are needled; sometimes spontaneous movements are induced. For example, when facial paralysis is treated, tremors of the orbicular muscle of the eye or of the facial and frontal muscles can occur when ear points are manipulated.

TREATMENT RESPONSES IN CHANNELS AND NETWORK VESSELS

A radiating sensation of soreness, numbness, or an electric feeling along one of the channels is sometimes felt when ear points are treated, particularly in the foot greater yáng bladder channel and in the foot yáng brightness stomach channel. For example, when sciatica is treated by needling Buttocks (MA-AH5) and Sciatic Nerve (MA-AH6), the needle sensation can radiate to the foot along the foot greater yáng bladder channel. This sensation is directly related to manipulation techniques. In general, stronger stimulation will induce stronger radiation of the needle sensation.

GENERALIZED TREATMENT RESPONSES

Some ear acupuncture patients will find that after treatments they have a boost in energy and immune function. Others may experience more vigorous gastrointestinal peristalsis. When dermal disorders are treated, cold or hot sensations on the skin are felt in some cases.

LIGHTNING–LIKE TREATMENT RESPONSE

This response is commonly seen in patients with acutely painful disorders, such as headache or toothache. Although the treatment sensation is quite harsh, when a lightening–like response is felt, the underlying pain usually disappears very quickly.

CHAIN RESPONSES

The treatment of one disorder with ear acupuncture can heal another disorder simultaneously. For example, with the relief of cough in treating bronchitis, dermal disorders in both lower limbs may be healed.

RESIDUAL RESPONSES

In some cases, the effect of treatment is not obvious at the completion of a course of therapy, but all manifestations greatly improve during the non-treatment period that follows. It is considered that ear acupuncture treatment stimulates the body to cure itself. If the disorder is not healed during the treatment period, perhaps because of a weak constitution or mild stimulation, the treatment nevertheless residually promotes the body's resistance to the disorder.

DESENSITIZED REACTIONS

In a portion of patients there will be good progress made by the first few treatments, yet after a period of time the patient's body becomes de-sensitized to the therapy, which results in later treatments making little or no effect. When it is seen that the patient is becoming desensitized, one should arrange for longer breaks between treatments. By allowing the ear points to fully rest and recover their sensitivity to stimulation, therapeutic effectiveness increases.

ABSENCE OF TREATMENT RESPONSE

If there are no discernible treatment responses to ear acupuncture treatments, the effect will not be very beneficial, so ear acupuncture should be discontinued.

NEGATIVE TREATMENT RESPONSES

In some cases, a patient's original complaint can be aggravated by ear acupuncture, such as with dizziness, headache, palpitations, and insomnia. This situation can be brought about by improper point selection, manipulation, or stimulation, or by the patient's mental state. Ear acupuncture should be discontinued for as long as negative treatment responses occur.

Management of Acupuncture Accidents

FAINTING

Fainting may be induced by ear acupuncture.

Causes

Weak constitution, mental stress, fear of pain, overstrain, hunger, profuse sweating, severe diarrhea or bleeding, strong stimulation.

Signs

During needling, especially during the time ear needles are retained, some patients will suddenly manifest listlessness, dizziness, oppression in the chest, palpitations, pale face, nausea, vomiting, cold limbs, and low blood pressure; in extreme situations there may be fainting, loss of consciousness, reversal cold of the four limbs, great and profuse sweating, and faint pulse verging on expiration.

Management

Stop treatment and withdraw all needles. Make the patient lie flat, loosen the clothing, and keep the body temperature warm. Sugar water or hot water can be given. Needling Subcortex (MA-AT1) and Adrenal Gland (MA-T) may be done in severe cases. A respiratory stimulant or cardiac tonic injected into some points can be used in severe cases, if necessary. Oxygen inhalation is commonly given.

Prevention

An explanation should be given before treating patients with mental stress. Patients with a history of fainting in response to acupuncture should lie down during treatment, and the treatment should be done using mild stimulation and just a few points. Patients who have overstrained or have strong hunger or thirst should take adequate rest and food before treatment. The practitioner should continuously observe the patient and treatment should cease for as long as any indications of fainting are manifest.

SKIN INFECTION

An infection may occur in the ear.

Causes

Sterilization of needles or of the skin at the treatment site is not strictly observed.

Signs

Redness, swelling, hot sensation, and pain in the affected area.

Management

Apply 2.5% iodine tincture, three times per day, together with ear acupressure at Adrenal Gland (MA-T), Ear Shén Mén (MA-TF1), Lung (MA-IC1), and External Ear (MA-L), once each day. Erythromycin ointment can be applied to affected areas. The lesions commonly heal in one to three days.

Prevention

All needles as well as the skin in the area to be treated should be thoroughly sterilized before treatment.

INFECTION OF AURICULAR CARTILAGE

Causes

Improper management of ear infection, or poor sterilization of needles.

Signs

Severe redness, swelling, hot sensation, and pain in affected areas that is accompanied by fever and chills.

Management

Use a 1000–2500G (gauss) magnetic pad covered with gauze with the poles placed in opposition in the affected area; fix it with an adhesive bandage using mild pressure. An antibiotic can also be used. Low temperature moxibustion can be applied to affected areas two or three times per day for 15 to 30 minutes each treatment until the inflammation is reduced. Purulent lesions cannot be managed with this method.

MANAGEMENT OF ABNORMAL SENSATIONS

Severe pain in the ear, palpitations, headache, difficulty in opening the mouth, coldness of the lower limbs, and numbness of the body can occur during ear acupuncture manipulations. These symptoms are generally caused by excessive manipulation at points like Adrenal Gland (MA-T), Sympathetic (MA-AH7), Endocrine (MA-IC3), Heart (MA-IC), and Internal Reproductive organs (MA-TF). Using only mild stimulation in these points will prevent the occurrence of such symptoms.

CHARACTERISTICS OF EAR POINT SELECTION AND PRINCIPLES OF PRESCRIPTION FORMATION

Characteristics of Ear Point Selection

The patient can either sit or lie down. The basis for ear point selection is that the precise location will be sensitive when pressed. The locations should be carefully determined because the size of ear points is smaller than that of body points.

Prescription Formation Principles

There are several principles for compiling prescriptions:

POINT SELECTION ACCORDING TO CORRESPONDING ORGANS OR AREAS

Examples of this include using Heart (MA-IC) for heart disorders, Stomach (MA-IC) for gastric disorder, Kidney (MA-SC) for chronic or acute nephritis or pyelonephritis, and Neck (MA-AH10), Shoulder (MA-SF4), Ankle (MA-AH2), and Hip (MA-AH4) for pain in the neck, shoulder, ankle, or hip, respectively.

POINT SELECTION ACCORDING TO TCM THEORY

For example, Lung (MA-IC1) may be used for dermal disorders because the lung governs skin. Eye (MA-L1) may be used for liver disorders because the liver opens at the eyes. Kidney (MA-SC) may be used for tinnitus and deafness because the kidney opens at the ears. Heart (MA-IC) may be used for insomnia because the heart governs the spirit light. Liver (MA-SC5) may be used for menstrual disorders because the foot reverting yīn liver channel travels along the medial side of the thigh, around the external genitals, and to the lower abdomen.

POINT SELECTION ACCORDING TO MODERN MEDICAL THEORY

Adrenal Gland (MA-T) can be used for low blood pressure, inflammation, allergic disorders, and rheumatoid arthritis because adrenocortical hormone (ACH) has anti-inflammatory, anti-allergic, and analgesic functions. Subcortex (MA-AT1) and Sympathetic (MA-AH7) are used for digestive tract ulcers that are caused by mental stress, melancholy, and overstrain related to functional disturbance of the sympathetic and vagus nerves. Pancreas/Gallbladder (MA-SC6), Endocrine (MA-IC3) and Central Rim (MA-AT) are used for diabetes, which is caused by a disturbance of endocrine functions.

POINT SELECTION ACCORDING TO POINT FUNCTIONS

Some ear points have their own functions. For example, Ear Shén Mén (MA-TF1) not only clears the mind and quiets the spirit but also serves as the primary point to relieve pain; it is used to treat almost all disorders with pain. Occiput (MA-AT) relieves dizziness, so it is used to treat dizziness and headaches that may be aspects of various disorders. Ear Apex (MA-H6) has anti-allergy, anti-inflammation, fever draining, spirit quieting, and blood pressure lowering effects, so it is used to treat allergic disorders, fever, insomnia, and hypertension.

POINT SELECTION ACCORDING TO CLINICAL EXPERIENCE

According to the clinical experience of many practitioners, Ear Shén Mén (MA-TF1) in combination with Occiput (MA-AT) quiets the spirit and relieves pain and so these points are used in treating insomnia and various pain disorders. Kidney (MA-SC), Spleen (MA-IC), Lung (MA-IC1), Triple Burner (MA-IC4), and Endocrine (MA-IC3) are often used to treat nephritis, ascites, and edema because the kidney governs water. Bladder (MA-SC8) is effective for treating diabetes insipidus, enuresis, and frequent urination because the bladder governs fluid storage.

The best therapeutic results come from knowing the general and specific natures of ear points, from finding points of positive reaction in regions of the ear that correspond to the illness, and as well from careful pattern identification and symptomatic point selection. When one also keeps in mind accumulating and applying clinical experience, one can fully develop the capacities of ear acupuncture.

CHAPTER TWO

THE EAR AND EAR POINTS AND AREAS

The ear is composed of three parts: the external ear, the middle ear, and the internal ear. The external ear includes the external auditory canal and the auricle. There are four prominences, three depressions, four notches, and one ear lobe on the anterior surface of the auricle (Figure 2.1).

• *Helix*: The curling rim of the most lateral border of the auricle, consisting of the helix root, the tubercle, and the helix cauda.

• *Helix root:* The transverse ridge of the helix continuing backward into the ear cavity.

• *Helix–lobe notch:* The depression between the helix and the posterior border of the ear lobe, at the lower border of the helix (the helix cauda).

• *Helix tubercle (Darwin's tubercle):* A tiny bump at the lateral–superior aspect of the helix, located anywhere between Wrist (MA-SF2) and Elbow (MA-SF3).

• *Helix Cauda:* The lower border of the helix where it meets the lobe.

• *Antihelix:* At the medial aspect of the helix, a Y-shaped protruding ridge that curves parallel to the helix. It is divided into three parts: superior antihelix crus, inferior antihelix crus, and body of the antihelix.

• *Tragus*: A curved flap in front of the auricle. There are two obvious prominences in the tragus: the upper apex of the tragus and the lower apex of the tragus.

• *Antitragus:* A small tubercle opposite to the tragus and superior to the upper part of the ear lobe.

• *Scaphoid fossa (also known as the scapha):* The narrow, curved depression between the helix and antihelix.

Anatomical Areas on the Anterior Surface of the Auricle

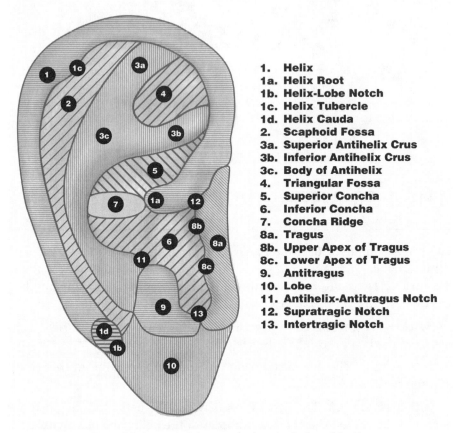

1. **Helix**
1a. **Helix Root**
1b. **Helix-Lobe Notch**
1c. **Helix Tubercle**
1d. **Helix Cauda**
2. **Scaphoid Fossa**
3a. **Superior Antihelix Crus**
3b. **Inferior Antihelix Crus**
3c. **Body of Antihelix**
4. **Triangular Fossa**
5. **Superior Concha**
6. **Inferior Concha**
7. **Concha Ridge**
8a. **Tragus**
8b. **Upper Apex of Tragus**
8c. **Lower Apex of Tragus**
9. **Antitragus**
10. **Lobe**
11. **Antihelix-Antitragus Notch**
12. **Supratragic Notch**
13. **Intertragic Notch**

Figure 2.1: Anatomical Areas on the Anterior Surface of the Ear

• *Triangular fossa*: The triangular depression between the two crusa of the antihelix.

• *Concha*: The depression encircled by the antitragus, the curving part of the antihelix, and the inferior antihelix crus. It consists of two parts: superior concha and inferior concha. The raised area of the concha posterior to the helix root is the concha ridge.

• *Lobe*: The lowest part of the auricle; it has no cartilage.

• *Supratragic notch*: The depression between the upper border of the tragus and the helix root.

• *Intertragic notch*: The depression between the tragus and the antitragus.

• *Antihelix–antitragus notch*: The depression between the antihelix and the antitragus.

Anatomical Areas on the Posterior Surface of the Auricle

There are three flat areas, five grooves, and four prominences on the posterior surface of the auricle (Figure 2.2).

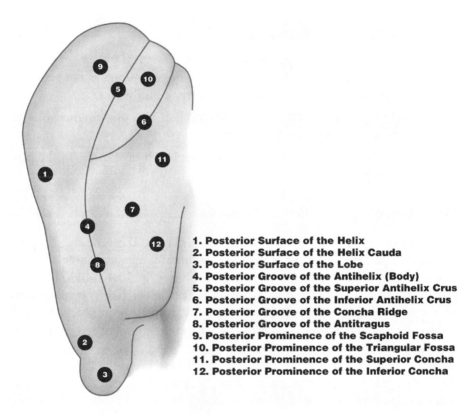

1. **Posterior Surface of the Helix**
2. **Posterior Surface of the Helix Cauda**
3. **Posterior Surface of the Lobe**
4. **Posterior Groove of the Antihelix (Body)**
5. **Posterior Groove of the Superior Antihelix Crus**
6. **Posterior Groove of the Inferior Antihelix Crus**
7. **Posterior Groove of the Concha Ridge**
8. **Posterior Groove of the Antitragus**
9. **Posterior Prominence of the Scaphoid Fossa**
10. **Posterior Prominence of the Triangular Fossa**
11. **Posterior Prominence of the Superior Concha**
12. **Posterior Prominence of the Inferior Concha**

Figure 2.2: Anatomical Areas on the Posterior Surface of the Ear

• *Posterior surface of the helix*: Lateral aspect of the helix from the helix curving forward, from the frontal aspect.

• *Posterior surface of the helix cauda*: The flat area between the posterior surfaces of the scaphoid fossa and ear lobe.

• *Posterior surface of the lobe*: The flat area that is the posterior surface of the lobe.

• *Posterior groove of antihelix body*: The groove in the posterior surface of the antihelix body (where the ear attaches).

• *Posterior groove of the superior antihelix crus*: The depression on the posterior surface of the superior antihelix crus.

• *Posterior groove of the inferior antihelix crus*: The depression on the posterior surface of the inferior antihelix crus.

• *Posterior groove of the concha ridge:* The depression on the posterior surface of the concha ridge.

• *Posterior groove of the antitragus*: The posterior surface of the antitragus.

• *Posterior prominence of the scaphoid fossa*: The prominence on the posterior surface of the scaphoid fossa.

• *Posterior prominence of the triangular fossa*: The prominence on the posterior surface of the triangular fossa, i.e., the prominence between the groove of the superior antihelix crus and inferior antihelix crus.

• *Posterior prominence of the superior concha*: The prominence on the posterior surface of the superior concha.

• *Posterior prominence of the inferior concha*: The prominence on the posterior surface of the inferior concha.

DEFINITION

Ear points are acupuncture points that are located on the ear; they are the linking places on the ear for the bowels and viscera, channels and network vessels, five offices, nine orifices, four limbs, and all bones. They are also the places where channel qì resides. Because ear points have a complex relationship with channels and network vessels, bowels and viscera, the nervous system, and body fluids, they can reflect on both physiological functions and pathological changes in the whole body by means of changes in color, appearance, and sensation. This is why practitioners can determine the location and property of a disorder by diagnosing the ear and can also treat the disorder by stimulating ear points.

DISTRIBUTION PATTERN AND CLASSIFICATION OF EAR POINTS

Pattern of Distribution

Ear points are distributed in a certain pattern. On the anterior–lateral surface of the ear, the distribution of ear points corresponds to an inverted human fetus, with the head downward, buttocks and legs upward, and chest and trunk in the middle (Figure 2.3). In addition, points distributed from top to bottom around the root of the helix are related to the digestive tract.

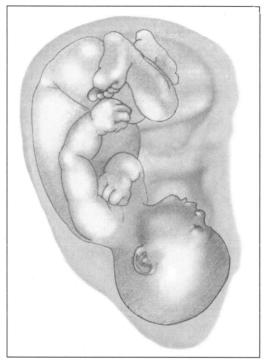

Figure 2.3: Anatomical Correspondence of the Ear and the Fetal Form

This is the general pattern of ear point distribution. However, practitioners should thoroughly understand that some points fall outside this pattern. The specific distribution is as follows:

POINTS LOCATED IN THE:	... ARE RELATED TO THE:
Ear lobe	Head and face
Scaphoid fossa	Upper limbs
Antihelix	Trunk
Inferior antihelix crus	Buttocks
Superior antihelix crus	Lower limbs
Helix root	Diaphragm
Superior concha	Abdomen
Inferior concha	Chest
Antitragus	Head and brain
Tragus	Adrenal gland and nose
Intertragic notch	Endocrine system
Triangular fossa	Pelvis

The majority of points are located on the anterior aspect of the ear. Figure 2.4 depicts the overall configuration of points and areas on the anterior aspect, and Figure 2.5 depicts the overall configuration of points and areas on the posterior aspect.

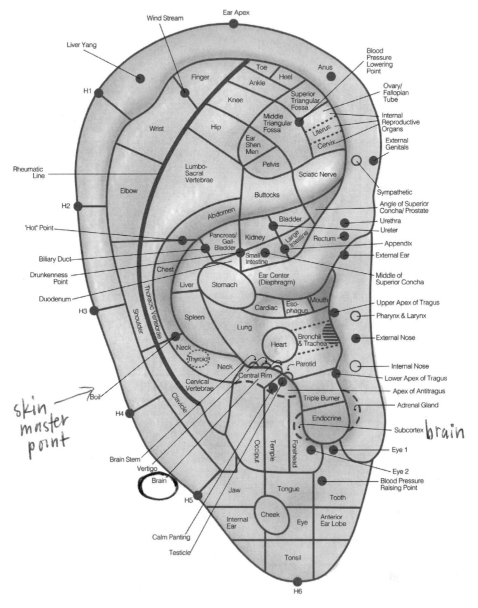

Figure 2.4: Points and Areas on the Anterior Aspect of the Ear

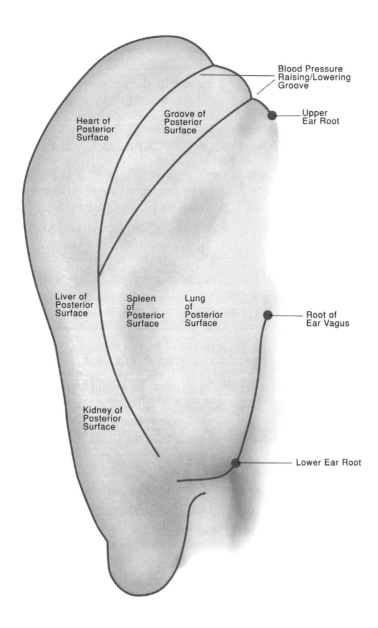

Figure 2.5: Points and Areas on the Posterior Aspect of the Ear

Classification of Ear Points and Areas

The Chinese Association of Acupuncture and Moxibustion was authorized by the World Health Organization to issue the *Standard Scheme of*

Ear Points in October of 1992. There are 90 points identified in this document. According to the naming characteristics, they are grouped into points that: (1) correspond to anatomical areas, (2) correspond to the five viscera and six bowels, (3) correspond to the nervous system, (4) correspond to the endocrine system, (5) are special points, and (6) are found on the posterior surface of the ear.

POINTS AND AREAS NAMED FOR CORRESPONDING ANATOMICAL REGIONS

Many ear points are regions of the ear that take their names from the anatomical regions to which they correspond. That is, when a specific organ or part is sick, a positive reaction in the ear will be seen in its corresponding region in the ear, and that region in the ear will be used to treat the diseased part. Here the corresponding region of the ear has a broad meaning of any point or region of the ear that becomes sensitive, or has a physical change, or some other positive reaction to a specific disease or disease in a specific region of the body. These points play an important role in ear diagnosis and are frequently primary selections when ear points are selected.

POINTS AND AREAS NAMED FOR THE FIVE VISCERA AND SIX BOWELS

The 11 areas named for the five viscera and six bowels include: Heart (MA-IC), Large Intestine (MA-SC4), Small Intestine (MA-SC2), Liver (MA-SC5), Spleen (MA-IC), Lung (MA-IC1), Kidney (MA-SC), Bladder (MA-SC8), Gallbladder (MA-SC6), Stomach (MA-IC), and Triple Burner (MA-IC4). Their names refer to TCM theories of the bowels and viscera, and the channels and network vessels. These ear areas individually (1) reflect diagnostic signs for specific disorders and (2) may treat multiple disorders. For example, according to TCM, the lung governs skin and body hair, it opens in the nose, and the throat is the door of the lung. So Lung (MA-IC1) is used to treat not only disorders related to the lung, but also disorders of the skin, nose, and throat. Bladder (MA-SC8) can be used to treat sciatica because the foot greater yáng bladder channel traverses the painful area. While there are just a few such areas, identifying them carefully is very important for ear diagnosis and treatment. In performing diagnosis, when one of these ear areas reflects a pathological change, this information should be incorporated into determining treatment by pattern identification.

POINTS AND AREAS NAMED FOR THE NERVOUS SYSTEM

Of the ear points and areas related to the nervous system, some points are named for corresponding parts of the nervous system, including Sympathetic (MA-AH7), Forehead (MA-AT), Temple (MA-AT), Occiput (MA-AT), and Sciatic Nerve (MA-AH6), while Ear Shén Mén (MA-TF1) and

Subcortex (MA-AT1) regulate excitement and inhibition of the cerebral cortex. In addition, Anterior Ear Lobe (MA-L) is used to treat neuroses, and Subcortex (MA-AT1) is an important point used to treat disorders of the nervous system. The proper utilization of these points can greatly increase the therapeutic effect of ear acupuncture.

POINTS AND AREAS NAMED FOR THE ENDOCRINE SYSTEM

There are eight aeas named for corresponding areas of the endocrine system: Endocrine (MA-IC3), Central Rim (MA-AT, *Yuán Zhōng*) (the corresponding area of the pituitary gland), Thyroid (MA-AH, *Jiǎ Zhuàng Xiàn*), Testicle (MA-AT, *Gāo Wán*), Ovary (MA-AT, *Luǎn Cháo*), Prostate/Angle of Superior Concha (MA-SC, *Qián Liè Xiàn*), Adrenal Gland (MA-T, *Shèng Shàng Xiàn*), and Pancreas/Gallbladder (MA-SC6). There are six other area that correspond to the endocrine glands. These points regulate physiological functions of the body by balancing secretions from endocrine glands, and physical and chemical factors.

Although the individual areas have correspondences to specific aspects of the endocrine system, in clinical practice it has been observed that ear point areas have mutually reinforcing and enhancing effects when the endocrine system is treated. Usually several points are used to accomplish the goal of regulating overall endocrine function. For example, amenorrhea can be treated with very strong effectiveness by using Endocrine (MA-IC3), Ovaries (MA-AT), Central Rim (MA-AT), and Internal Reproductive Organs (MA-TF). The combination of Endocrine (MA-IC3), Pancreas/Gallbladder (MA- SC6), and Central Rim (MA-AT) can quickly improve certain symptoms, such as dry mouth, poor appetite, and numbness and listlessness in diabetic patients, which demonstrates that they can effectively regulate insulin metabolism.

SPECIAL POINTS

Special ear points are those that have specific functions in diagnosis and treatment. Generally speaking, a positive reaction at one point can reflect different disorders, and one disorder can lead to positive reactions at several points. These phenomena must be interpreted with theoretical knowledge from TCM and/or modern biomedicine. However, a positive reaction at one of the special ear points indicates a very specific disorder. For example, Wind Stream (MA-SF) is an important point indicating an allergic constitution and allergic disorders, and Blood Pressure Raising (MA-PS) can be used to diagnose and treat low blood pressure. These points can clarify diagnosis and treatment in some cases of the diseases to which they pertain.

Additionally there are a number of points and areas that are named by their appearance and location in the ear, such as Ear Apex (MA-H6), Apex of Tragus (MA-T2), and Helix 1-6 (MA-H 1-6). Helix 1-6 is the region from the lower border of the helix tubercle to the midpoint of the lower border of the lobule.

POINTS AND AREAS ON THE POSTERIOR SURFACE

There are three points and six areas altogether on the posterior surface of the ear: Heart of Posterior Surface (MA-PS, *Ěr Bèi Xīn*), Liver of Posterior Surface (MA-PS, *Ěr Bèi Gān*), Spleen of Posterior Surface (MA-PS, *Ěr Bèi Pí*), Lung of Posterior Surface (MA-PS, *Ěr Bèi Fèi*), Kidney of Posterior Surface (MA-PS, *Ěr Bèi Shèn*), Groove of Posterior Surface (MA-PS, *Ěr Bèi Gōu*), Upper Ear Root (MA-PS, *Shàng Ěr Gēn*), Root of Ear Vagus (MA-PS, *Ěr Mí Gēn*), and Lower Ear Root (MA-PS, *Xià Ěr Gēn*).

The first five points share the same anatomical correspondence and physiological functions with those having the same names on the anterior surface.

STANDARD NAMES, LOCATIONS, AND INDICATIONS ASSOCIATED WITH EAR POINTS AND AREAS

Helix Points and Areas (MA-H)

EAR CENTER (MA-H1)

> **Location:** On the helix root.
> **Functions:** Resolve tetany and check hiccoughs; downbear counterflow stomach qì and check vomiting; rectify the blood and dispel wind.
> **Indications:** Hiccoughs, vomiting due to spasm of diaphragm and other reasons; all diseases due to blood vacuity, blood stasis, and blood heat; bleeding such as hemoptysis, flooding and spotting.

RECTUM (MA-H2)

> **Location:** At the end of the helix near the supratragic notch, level with Large Intestine (MA-SC4).
> **Functions:** Free the stool and check diarrhea. This point regulates both of these rectal functions.
> **Indications:** Constipation, diarrhea, prolapse of the rectum, hemorrhoid, tenesmus occurring in dysentery.

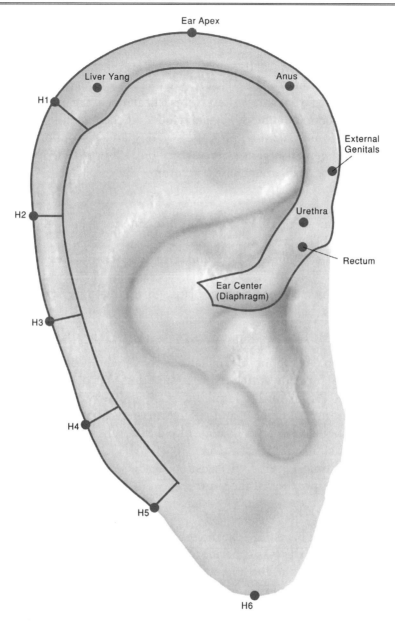

Figure 2.6: Points and Areas on the Helix of the Ear

URETHRA (MA-H3)

Location: At the helix, superior to Rectum (MA-H2), at the level of the ureter point between the Kidney and Bladder areas.

Functions: Clear heat and disinhibit urine.

Indications: Frequent, urgent, and painful urination, frequent urination at night, retention of urine.

EXTERNAL GENITALS (MA-H4)

Location: At the helix, superior to Urethra (MA-H3), level with Sympathetic (MA-AH7).

Functions: Clear and drain damp heat from the liver and gall-bladder; cool blood, dispel wind, and check itching.

Indications: Balanitis, orchitis, swelling and discomfort of external genital organs after surgery on fallopian tube, pruritus of vulva, and eczema of the scrotum.

ANUS (MA-H5)

Location: At the helix, opposite the anterior rim of the superior antihelix crus.

Functions: Quicken the blood, free the network vessels and relieve pain.

Indications: Hemorrhoid, prolapse of the rectum, pruritus of the anus.

EAR APEX (MA-H6)

Location: At the top of the helix, opposite the posterior border of the superior antihelix crus (superior root of antihelix). Fold the ear forward to locate the point at the crease of the fold.

Functions: Clear heat and resolve toxins; calm the liver and extinguish liver wind; cool blood and relieve itching; disperse swelling and relieve pain.

Indications: Fever, hypertension, headache, dizziness, eye disorders, pruritus of the skin.

LIVER YÁNG (MA-H)

Location: This point is at the tubercle of the helix, a tiny notch on the helix that is superior to the wrist area.

Functions: Calm the liver and subdue yáng, drain fire and resolve toxins.

Indications: Headache, dizziness, bloodshot eyes, hypertension, acute and chronic hepatitis, and rib-side pain and distention due to ascendant hyperactivity of liver yáng.

HELIX 1-6 (H-1, H-2, H-3, H-4, H-5, H-6)

Location: The helix area from the lower border of the helix tubercle to the midpoint of the lower border of the ear lobe is divided into five equal parts (six points). The points marking the divisions are named H-1, H-2, H-3, H-4, H-5, and H-6, respectively. To locate these clinically, mark the lower border of the helix tubercle as H-1 and mark H-6 (the lowest point of the ear lobe). Divide the area between these to into five equal parts. The remaining H- points are at the division lines.

Functions: Clear heat and resolve toxins; disperse swelling and relieve pain.

Indications: Fever, tonsillitis, sore throat, upper respiratory tract infection.

Scaphoid Fossa (Scapha) Points and Areas (MA-SF)

FINGER (MA-SF1)

Location: Dividing the scapha into five parts from top to bottom, this area is the first portion of the scapha.

Functions: Quicken the blood and dispel wind; free the network vessels and relieve pain.

Indications: Sprain and contusion of finger joints, dermal disorders, profuse sweating, pain and numbness of fingers due to cervical spondylopathy.

WRIST (MA-SF2)

Location: This area is the second portion of the scapha.

Functions: Quicken the blood and dispel wind; free the network vessels and relieve pain.

Indications: Sprain and contusion of wrist, allergic dermal disorders.

WIND STREAM (WIND RAVINE) (MA-SF)

Location: This is the only point on the scapha, and is located midway between Finger (MA-SF1) and Wrist (MA-SF2).

Functions: Quicken the blood and dispel wind; free the network vessels and relieve pain.

Indications: Urticaria, pruritus and allergic dermatitis, rhinallergosis.

ELBOW (MA-SF3)

Location: This area is the third portion of the scapha.

Functions: Quicken the blood and dispel wind; free the network vessels and relieve pain.

Indications: External humeral epicondylitis and pain in the elbow.

SHOULDER (MA-SF4)

Location: This area is the fourth section of the scapha.

Functions: Quicken the blood and dispel wind; free the network vessels and relieve pain.

Indications: Periarthritis of the shoulder joint, crick in the neck, subacromial bursitis, and pain in the shoulders.

CLAVICLE (MA-SF5)

Location: This area is the fifth portion of the scapha.

Functions: Dispel wind, free the network vessels, and relieve pain.

Indications: Shoulder pain resulting from any cause.

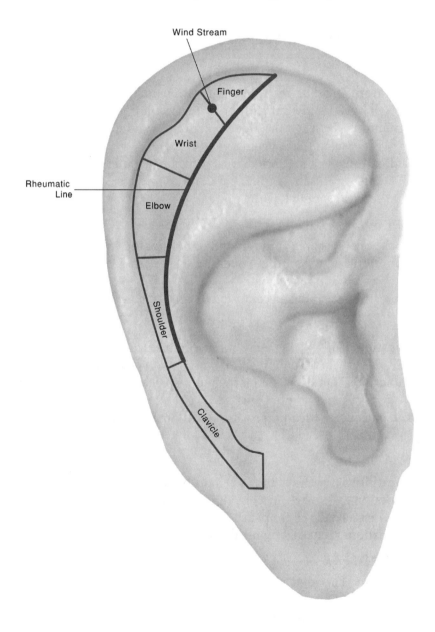

Figure 2.7: Points and Areas on the Scaphoid Fossa of the Ear

Antihelix Points and Areas (MA-AH)

TOE (MA-AH)

Location: Posterior upper corner of the superior antihelix crus, near the ear apex.

Functions: Quicken the blood and dispel wind; reduce swelling and relieve pain.

Indications: Paronychia and pain in toes, Raynaud's syndrome, and erythromelalgia.

HEEL (MA-AH1)

Location: Anterior upper corner of superior antihelix crus, near the upper end of the triangular fossa.

Functions: Strengthen sinew and invigorate bone, quicken the blood and dispel wind.

Indications: Pain in heels.

ANKLE (MA-AH2)

Location: Area between Heel (MA-AH1) and Knee (MA-AH3).

Functions: Strengthen sinew and invigorate bone, quicken the blood and dispel wind, reduce swelling and relieve pain.

Indications: Sprain and contusion of ankle joint, arthritis in ankle joint.

KNEE (MA-AH3)

Location: The middle third of the superior antihelix crus.

Functions: Dispel wind, eliminate damp, free the network vessels, and relieve pain.

Indications: Pain in knee joint and limited range of motion of lower extremities seen in various disorders.

HIP (MA-AH4)

Location: The lower third of the superior antihelix crus.

Functions: Quicken the blood; free the network vessels, dispel wind, and relieve pain.

Indications: Sciatica and pain in the lumbosacral area and around the hip joint.

BUTTOCKS (MA-AH5)

Location: The posterior third of the inferior antihelix crus.

Functions: Quicken the blood and dispel wind; free the network vessels and relieve pain.

Indications: Sciatica, pain in buttocks and sacral area.

SCIATIC NERVE (MA-AH6)

Location: The anterior two-thirds of the inferior antihelix crus.

Functions: Strengthen sinew and invigorate bone, quicken the blood and free the network vessels, reduce swelling and relieve pain.

Indications: Sciatica, flaccidity of lower limbs, painful impediment, paralysis.

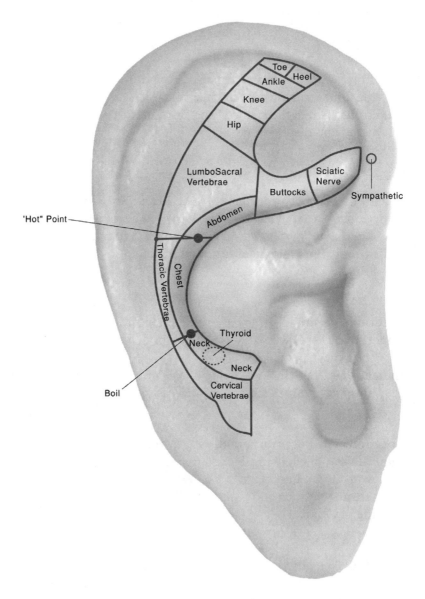

Figure 2.8: Points on the Antihelix of the Ear

SYMPATHETIC (MA-AH7)

Location: A point on the interior aspect at the junction of the antihelix and helix, level with sciatic nerve (MA-AH6). Clinically, the point is taped in the antihelix part, as close as possible to the groove.

Functions: Regulate sympathetic and parasympathetic nervous systems; relieve spasm of smooth muscles; regulate vascular contraction and relieve pain in internal organs.

Indications: Various disorders caused by disturbance of autonomic nervous system, such as insomnia, profuse sweating, dysfunction of sympathetic nerves, colic of internal organs, sexual dysfunction, angina pectoris, pulseless syndrome, thrombophlebitis and Raynaud's syndrome.

LUMBOSACRAL VERTEBRAE (MA-AH)

Location: Upper one-third of the antihelix body. The line from the intertragic notch to the antihelix crus is divided into three parts. The upper third is Lumbosacral Vertebrae.

Functions: Strengthen the lumbus and fortify kidney; free and quicken the channels and network vessels; disperse swelling and relieve pain.

Indications: Pain in lumbosacral areas and limited range of motion of lower limbs found in various disorders such as sprain and contusion of lumbosacral vertebrae, hyperosteogeny of lumbosacral vertebrae, lumbar muscle strain, rheumatoid arthritis, pyelitis, and nephrolithiasis.

ABDOMEN (MA-AH)

Location: The upper part of the antihelix body, at the anterior aspect of Lumbosacral Vertebrae (MA-AH), near the rim of the scapha.

Functions: Free the channels and network vessels; soften muscle and resolve tetany; disperse swelling and relieve pain.

Indications: Acute or chronic colitis, abdominal pain, constipation, dysmenorrhea, pain in lower abdomen after childbirth, muscular pain after surgery, loss of weight.

THORACIC VERTEBRAE (MA-AH9)

Location: The middle one-third of the antihelix body.

Functions: Quicken the channels and network vessels; disperse swelling and relieve pain.

Indications: Disorders in thoracic vertebrae, pain in the back and chest due to sprain and contusion, mastitis.

CHEST (MA-AH11)

Location: The middle part of the antihelix at the anterior aspect of Thoracic Vertebrae (MA-AH9), near the rim of the scapha.

Functions: Quicken the channels and network vessels; disperse swelling and relieve pain.

Indications: Pain in chest and hypochondrium, oppression in the chest, mastitis, and disorders in the thoracic cavity.

CERVICAL VERTEBRAE (MA-AH8)

Location: On the antihelix body, the line from the intertragic notch to the bifurcation of the superior antihelix crus and the inferior antihelix crus is divided into three parts. The lowest third is Cervial Vertebrae (MA-AH8).

Functions: Strengthen tendons and bones; free the network vessels and relieve pain.

Indications: Cervical spondylopathy, neck pain from all causes (such as crick in the neck), rheumatoid arthritis, spondylitis, hypothyroidism and hyperthyroidism.

NECK (MA-AH10)

Location: The lower part of the antihelix at the anterior aspect of Cervical Vertebrae (MA-AH8), near the border of scapha.

Functions: Quicken the channels and network vessels; relieve pain.

Indications: Cervical spondylopathy, sprain and contusion of the neck, stiff neck, hypothyroidism, and hyperthyroidism.

Triangular Fossa Points and Areas (MA-TF)

The triangular fossa is considered to be representative of the uterus.

EAR SHÉN MÉN (MA-TF1)

Location: On the triangular fossa at the superior aspect of the bifurcating point of the superior antihelix crus and the inferior antihelix crus.

Functions: Quiet the spirit; resolve tetany and relieve pain; clear heat and resolve toxins; dispel wind and relieve itching.

Indications: Insomnia, dream-disturbed sleep, dysphoria, hysteria, various inflammations and pain occurring in the face, head, body and internal organs; neuralgia, hypertension, and allergic disorders.

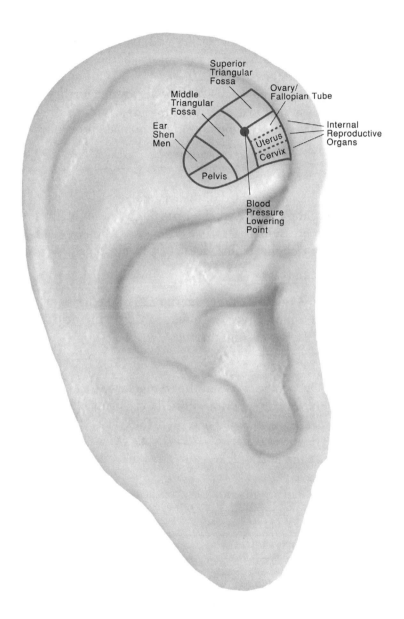

Figure 2.9: Points and Areas on the Triangular Fossa of the Ear

INTERNAL REPRODUCTIVE ORGANS (MA-TF)

Location: The inferior half of the anterior third of the triangular fossa. The upper portion of this area relates to the adnexa (*Fù Jiàng*), the ovaries and fallopian tubes. The middle portion corresponds to the uterus, and the lower portion to the cervix (*Gōng Jǐng*).

Functions: Supplement the kidney and boost the essence; regulate menstruation and check vaginal discharge; free the network vessels and relieve pain.

Indications: Irregular menstrual cycle, dysmenorrhea, amenorrhea, dysfunctional uterine bleeding, profuse vaginal discharge, pelvic inflammation, impotence, prostatitis, sexual dysfunction.

MIDDLE TRIANGULAR FOSSA (MA-TF)

Location: The middle third of the triangular fossa.

Functions: Stop cough and calm panting; soothe the liver and resolve depression.

Indications: Cough, asthma, acute or chronic hepatitis.

SUPERIOR TRIANGULAR FOSSA (MA-TF)

Location: Superior 1/2 of the anterior 1/3 of the triangular fossa.

Functions: Calm the liver and subdue yáng; extinguish wind.

Indications: Hypertension, dizziness.

PELVIS (MA-TF)

Location: The posterior 1/3 of the triangular fossa, at the bifurcating point of the superior antihelix crus and inferior antihelix crus, is shared by Ear Shén Mén (MA-TF1) and Pelvis (MA-TF). The lower (inferior) 1/2 is Pelvis (MA-TF).

Functions: Free and quicken the channels and network vessels; and relieve pain.

Indications: Pelvic inflammation, prostatitis, pain in lower abdomen and dysmenorrhea.

Tragus points (MA-T)

EXTERNAL NOSE (MA-T1)

Location: Anterior to middle of the lateral aspect of the tragus, on the outer surface.

Functions: Dispel stasis and free the network vessels; course wind and relieve pain.

Indications: Nasal disorders such as rhinallergosis.

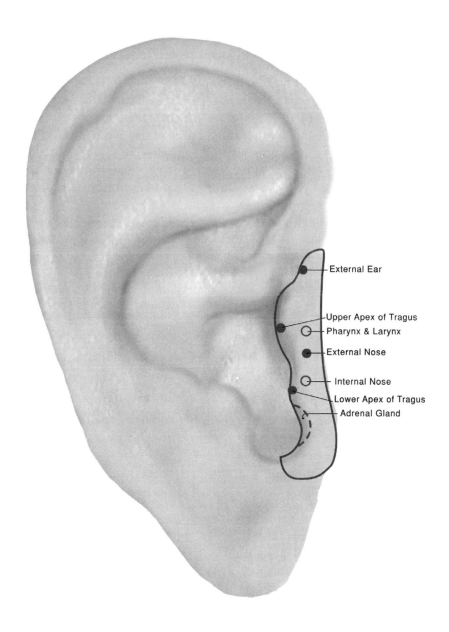

Figure 2.10: Points and Areas on the Tragus of the Ear

LOWER APEX OF TRAGUS (MA-T2)

Location: Tip of the inferior prominence of the tragus. (Some texts indicate an Upper Apex of Tragus and a Lower Apex of Tragus, the upper being the upper prominence and the lower being the lower prominence. Here we refer to the Lower Apex of Tragus.)

Functions: Clear heat and resolve toxins, quiet the spirit and relieve pain.

Indications: Fever and toothache as seen in various disorders.

ADRENAL GLAND (MA-T)

Location: Inferior to the lower apex of the tragus, level with Endocrine (MA-IC3) on medial (inner) side.

Functions: Regulate function of adrenal gland and adrenocortical hormones; anti-inflammatory; disperse swelling; treat allergic disorders and rheumatoid arthritis; regulate functions of the cardiovascular system and excite the respiratory aspect of the central nervous system.

Indications: High fever, mild fever, rheumatoid arthritis, mumps, cough, asthma, pruritis, hypertension, pulseless syndrome, coma, angitis.

PHARYNX AND LARYNX (MA-T3)

Location: The upper half of the medial (inner) surface of the tragus.

Functions: Clear heat and resolve toxins; disperse swelling and relieve pain.

Indications: Acute or chronic pharyngitis, tonsillitis, loss of voice, bronchitis.

INTERNAL NOSE (MA-T)

Location: The lower half of the inner surface of the tragus.

Functions: Course wind and resolve the exterior; free and disinhibit the nose.

Indications: Common cold, rhinitis, nasosinusitis, nasal bleeding.

EXTERNAL EAR (MA-T)

Location: Superior to the supratragic notch, near the helix, inferior to Rectum (MA-H2).

Functions: Dispel stasis and free the network vessels.

Indications: Inflammation of external auditory canal, otitis media, tinnitus.

Antitragus points (MA-AT)

APEX OF ANTITRAGUS (MA-AT)

Location: Apex of antitragus. According to the WHO international standards schema, Apex of Antitragus includes *Píng Chuǎn* (Calm Panting), *Sāi Xiàn* (Parotid), and *Gǎo Wán* (Testicle).[4] Parotid is located inside the line of the antitragus. Testicle is

---

[4] See footnote discussion on p. 162.

located by visualizing a line running diagonally and posteriorly, a little off the prominence of the apex on the anterior aspect. Calm Panting is located along the same diagonal line and about the same distance from Testicle as Testicle is from Parotid.

Functions: Stop cough and calm panting; course wind and free the network vessels.

Indications: Cough, asthma, difficult respiration, mumps, orchitis.

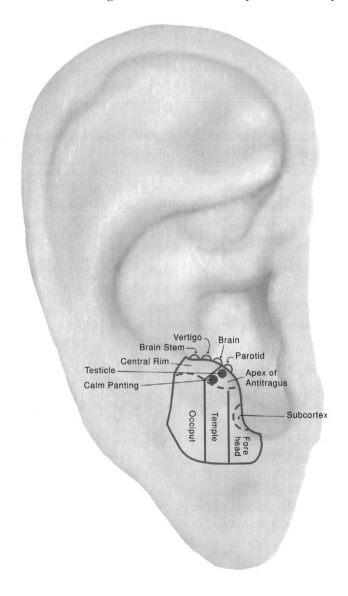

Figure 2.11: Points and Areas on the Antitragus of the Ear

CENTRAL RIM (MA-AT)

Location: Along the upper line of the antitragus, posterior to the Apex of Antitragus. There is a 1 cm curve above and inside the Central Rim. This area includes the Brain Stem (upper part), Vertigo (middle part), and Brain (lower part). The lowest part is level with the tragal point Internal Nose (MA-T).

Functions: Regulate functions of brain stem and pituitary gland; boost the brain and quiet the spirit.

Indications: Cerebritis, post-concussion syndrome, maldevelopment of the brain, dizziness, dysmenorrhea, dysfunctional uterine bleeding.

OCCIPUT (MA-AT)

Location: Posterior-superior corner of the lateral aspect of the antitragus.

Functions: Clear heat and extinguish wind; quiet the spirit; nourish the liver and brighten the eyes.

Indications: Dizziness and headache due to insufficiency of blood in the brain; motion sickness; convulsions, stiff neck and opisthotonus seen in cerebritis and traumatic brain injury; blurred vision, myopia, and cataract.

TEMPLE (MA-AT)

Location: Middle of the lateral aspect of the antitragus.

Functions: Course and disinhibit the liver and gallbladder; free the network vessels and relieve pain.

Indications: Headache, migraine and drowsiness.

FOREHEAD (MA-AT)

Location: Anterior-interior corner of the lateral aspect of the antitragus.

Functions: Quiet the spirit; free the network vessels and relieve pain.

Indications: Headache, dizziness, insomnia, rhinitis, nasosinusitis, myopia.

SUBCORTEX (MA-AT1)

Location: At the interior aspect of the antitragus, level with inferior concha area Endocrine (MA-IC3), on the lateral side. To locate, pull down on the antitragus or lobe; use an ear probe to locate the sensitive spot.

Functions: Regulate excitation and inhibition functions of the cerebral cortex; quiet the spirit; relieve pain; stop vomiting and secure desertion.

Indications: Insomnia, dream-disturbed sleep, forgetfulness, protracted inflammation, pain, vomiting, hiccoughs, headache, hysterical paralysis, pseudomyopia, shock.

Inferior Concha Points (MA-IC)

HEART (MA-IC)

Location: At the center of the inferior concha, below the terminus of the helix root.

Functions: Regulate functions of the cardiovascular and central nervous systems; settle the heart and quiet the spirit; regulate and harmonize the blood; clear the heart and drain fire.

Indications: Arrhythmia, angina pectoris, hypertension; neurosis, mental disorders, pharyngitis, loss of voice.

LUNG (MA-IC1)

Location: Around the center of the inferior concha. The anterior portion of the lung area level with Heart (MA-IC) is Bronchii/Trachea (MA-IC2) (qì guǎn).

Functions: Move qì and quicken the blood; stop cough and calm panting; disinhibit water and free the stool.

Indications: Acute or chronic bronchitis, asthma, pain in the chest; common cold; rhinitis, pharyngitis, night sweats, spontaneous sweating; urticaria, eczema, acne; constipation, diuresis, edema.

BRONCHII/TRACHEA (MA-IC2)

Location: The inferior concha between the opening of the external auditory canal and Heart (MA-IC).

Functions: Perfuse the lung and disinhibit qì; stop cough and dispel phlegm.

Indications: Acute or chronic bronchitis, cough, asthma, pharyngitis, common cold.

SPLEEN (MA-IC)

Location: Posterior-superior aspect of the inferior concha, posterior to Lung (MA-IC1).

Functions: Fortify the spleen and harmonize the stomach; boost qì and engender flesh.

Indications: Abdominal pain, distention in abdomen, diarrhea, stools retaining blood, epistaxis; atrophy, progressive myodystrophy; prolapse of the rectum and uterus.

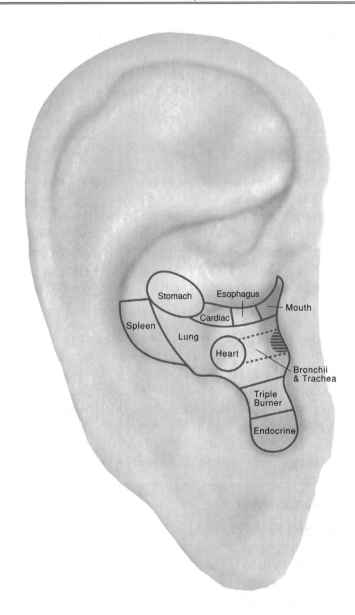

Figure 2.12: Points and Areas on the Inferior Concha

ENDOCRINE (MA-IC3)

Location: Fundus of inferior concha, in the intertragic notch.

Functions: Regulate functions of the endocrine system; anti-inflammatory, anti-allergy, and anti-rheumatoid arthritis.

Indications: Hyperthyroidism, obesity, irregular menstrual cycle, dysmenorrhea, amenorrhea, premenstrual syndrome, climacteric syndrome, prostatitis, seminal emission, sterility, urticaria, rhinallergosis, rheumatoid arthritis.

TRIPLE BURNER (SĀN JIĀO) (MA-IC4)

Location: Fundus of inferior concha, superior to Endocrine (MA-IC3) in the intertragic notch.

Functions: Diffuse the qì dynamic; free and regulate waterways.

Indications: Edema, diuresis, deafness, tinnitus, painful impediment.

MOUTH (MA-IC5)

Location: Anterior third of the upper portion of the inferior concha, posterior to the supratragal notch.

Functions: Dispel stasis and free the network vessels; relieve pain; stop cough.

Indications: Disorders occurring in mouth and throat such as ulcers, pharyngitis; bronchitis, tracheitis.

ESOPHAGUS (MA-IC6)

Location: Middle third of the upper portion of the inferior concha, between Mouth (MA-IC5) and Cardiac (MA-IC7).

Functions: Loosen the chest and disinhibit the diaphragm.

Indications: Inflammation of esophagus, oppression in the chest, difficult respiration.

CARDIAC (MA-IC7)

Location: Posterior third of the upper portion of the inferior concha, inferior to the helix root.

Functions: Quicken qì; resolve tetany and relieve pain.

Indications: Pain in upper abdomen, nausea, vomiting, oppression in the chest, poor appetite, distention of upper abdomen.

STOMACH (MA-IC)

Location: Posterior to the helix root, on the concha ridge.

Functions: Harmonize the stomach and downbear counterflow; resolve tetany and relieve pain.

Indications: Gastric ulcer, gastritis, maldigestion, hiccoughs, vomiting, headache, toothache.

Superior Concha Points (MA-SC)

DUODENUM (MA-SC1)

Location: Superior concha, the superior and posterior aspect of the helix root.

Functions: Resolve tetany and relieve pain.

Indications: Duodenal ulcer, cholelithiasis, cholecystitis, pyloric spasm.

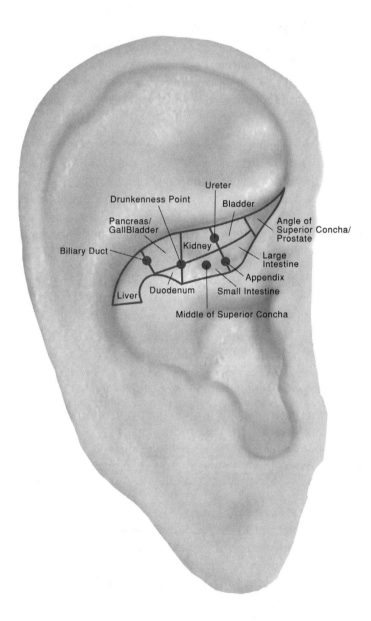

Figure 2.13: Points and Areas on the Superior Concha of the Ear

SMALL INTESTINE (MA-SC2)

Location: On the superior concha at superior and middle aspect of the helix root.

Functions: Disperse accumulations and transform food.

Indications: Maldigestion, abdominal distention, diarrhea, sore throat, sores in mouth. This is also a supplementary point for treating arrhythmia.

APPENDIX (MA-SC3)

Location: A point on the superior concha, between Large Intestine (MA-SC4) and Small Intestine (MA-SC2).
Functions: Dispel stasis and free the network vessels; resolve tetany and relieve pain.
Indications: Appendicitis, loose stools.

LARGE INTESTINE (MA-SC4)

Location: Superior concha, anterior and superior to the helix root.
Functions: Dispel wind, clear heat, and free the bowels.
Indications: Loose stools, constipation, cough, toothache, acne.

LIVER (MA-SC5)

Location: Posterior portion of the lower aspect of the superior concha, anterior to Chest (MA-AH11) and superior to Spleen (MA-IC).
Functions: Course the liver and rectify qì; brighten the eyes and extinguish wind.
Indications: Acute or chronic hepatitis, cholecystitis, cholelithiasis, distention and pain in the upper abdomen, belching, acid regurgitation; dizziness, convulsion, hemiparesis; myopia, sty, and acute conjunctivitis.

PANCREAS/GALLBLADDER (MA-SC6)

Location: Superior concha, between Liver (MA-SC5) and Kidney (MA-SC).
Functions: Course and disinhibit the liver and gallbladder; free the network vessels and relieve pain.
Indications: Cholecystitis, cholelithiasis, parasitic diseases of the biliary tract; acute or chronic pancreatitis; migraine, deafness, and tinnitus.

KIDNEY (MA-SC)

Location: Superior concha, inferior to Buttocks (MA-AH5) and posterior to and level with Bladder (MA-SC8).
Functions: Supplement kidney and boost essence; strengthen lumbus and invigorate bones.
Indications: Disorders of urinary and reproductive systems such as nephritis, cystitis, impotence, seminal emission; dysmenorrhea, amenorrhea; deafness, tinnitus, retardation of hearing, loss of hair; disorders of the nervous system such as poor development of the brain, headache, spinal retrograde degeneration, pain in lumbus, rheumatoid arthritis, chronic diarrhea, frequent urination at night, bedwetting.

URETER (MA-SC7)

Location: A point on the upper aspect of the superior concha between Kidney (MA-SC) and Bladder (MA-SC8).

Functions: Clear heat, disinhibit urine and free strangury.

Indications: Urinary infection, colic due to calculus in ureter.

BLADDER (MA-SC8)

Location: An area on the upper aspect of the superior concha between Kidney (MA-SC) and Angle of Superior Concha/Prostate (MA-SC).

Functions: Clear heat and disinhibit urine; free the network vessels and relieve pain.

Indications: Acute cystitis, pyelonephritis, prostatitis, bedwetting, urine retention, urinary incontinence; headache, pain in lumbar and spinal areas, sciatica.

MIDDLE OF SUPERIOR CONCHA (MA-SC)

Location: At the center of the superior concha, a point in the Small Intestine area.

Functions: Regulate flow of qì and relieve pain.

Indications: Pain around umbilicus, abdominal pain, dysmenorrhea, parasitic diseases of biliary tract, prostatitis, calculus of urinary system.

PROSTATE/ANGLE OF SUPERIOR CONCHA (MA-SC)

Location: At the narrow upper angle of the superior concha.

Functions: Treat prostate disorders.

Indications: Prostate disorders including prostatitis, urethritis, UTI, prostatic hypertrophy, and prostate cancer.

Lobe points (MA-L)

At the ear lobe, draw three proportional horizontal lines from the lower border of the cartilage of the intertragic notch to the inferior rim of the ear lobe and another two vertical and proportional lines from the second horizontal line. This divides the ear lobe into nine regions from front to back and from top to bottom.

It is worth noting that there are two points above regions 1 and 2 on the lobe. The anterior point is named Eye 1 and the posterior point is named Eye 2. They are used for all kinds of eye disorders.

EYE (MA-L)

Location: Fifth region of ear lobe.

Functions: Clear the liver, drain fire, and brighten the eyes.

Indications: Acute conjunctivitis, retinitis, sty, pseudomyopia, electric ophthalmia.

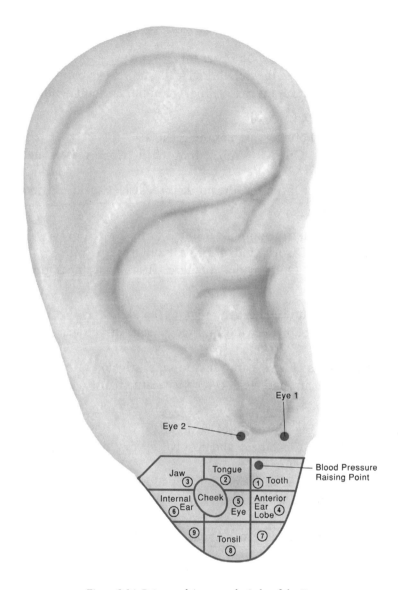

Figure 2.14: Points and Areas on the Lobe of the Ear

TOOTH (MA-L)

Location: First region of ear lobe.

Functions: Nourish the liver and brighten the eyes.

Indications: Glaucoma, retinitis, sty, optic atrophy, iridocyclitis, myopia.

TONGUE (MA-L)

Location: Second region of ear lobe.

Functions: Clear heat and resolve toxins; dispel stasis and free the network vessels.

Indications: Inflammation of the mouth and tongue.

JAW (MA-L)

Location: Third region of ear lobe.
Functions: Free the network vessels and relieve pain.
Indications: Toothache, temporomandibular joint syndrome.

ANTERIOR EAR LOBE (MA-L)

Location: Fourth region of the ear lobe.
Functions: Quiet the spirit; free the network vessels and relieve pain.
Indications: Insomnia, dream-disturbed sleep, neurosis, toothache.

INTERNAL EAR (MA-L)

Location: Sixth region of ear lobe.
Functions: Dispel wind, clear heat and free the orifice.
Indications: Otitis media, Menière's disease, deafness, tinnitus.

CHEEK (MA-L)

Location: Midway between regions 5 and 6.
Functions: Course wind and clear heat; dispel stasis and relieve pain.
Indications: Facial paralysis, mumps, trigeminal neuralgia, acne, chloasma, and facial cosmetic treatments.

TONSIL (MA-L)

Location: Eighth region of ear lobe.
Functions: Clear heat and resolve toxins; disperse swelling and relieve pain.
Indications: Acute or chronic tonsillitis, sore throat, fever found in various disorders.

Posterior Surface Points and Areas (MA-PS)

HEART OF POSTERIOR SURFACE (MA-PS)

Location: Upper part of the back of the ear.
Functions: Nourish the heart and quiet the spirit.
Indications: Palpitations, insomnia, dream-disturbed sleep, headache.

LUNG OF POSTERIOR SURFACE (MA-PS)

Location: From the area of Spleen of Posterior Surface (MA-PS) to the Lower Ear Root.
Functions: Perfuse the lung and disinhibit qì; stop cough and calm panting.
Indications: Tracheitis, bronchitis, bronchial asthma, pruritus.

SPLEEN OF POSTERIOR SURFACE (MA-PS)

Location: The posterior ear, in the area where the helix root terminates (anterior to Lung of Posterior Surface).

Functions: Fortify the spleen and harmonize the stomach.

Indications: Gastritis, pain and distention of abdomen, maldigestion, poor appetite as seen in gastroduodenal ulcer.

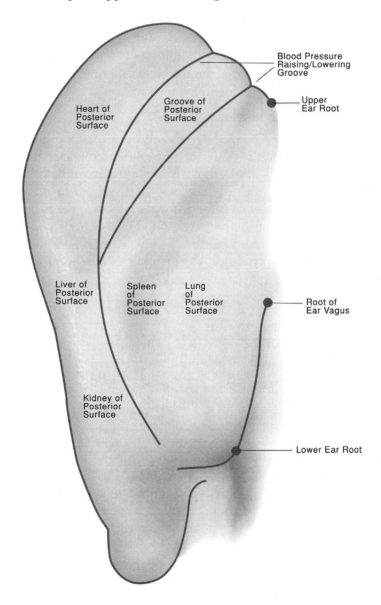

Figure 2.15: Points and Areas on the Posterior Surface of the Ear

LIVER OF POSTERIOR SURFACE (MA-PS)

Location: From Spleen of Posterior Surface (MA-PS) to the area of the helix.

Functions: Course the liver and disinhibit the gallbladder.

Indications: Cholecystitis, cholelithiasis, pain in upper abdomen, distention in hypochondrium, eye disorders.

KIDNEY OF POSTERIOR SURFACE (MA-PS)

Location: Lower part of the back of the ear.

Functions: Supplement the kidney and boost essence.

Indications: Dizziness, headache, dysphoria, insomnia, dream-disturbed sleep due to kidney vacuity.

GROOVE OF POSTERIOR SURFACE (MA-PS)

Location: In a Y-shaped depression on the back of the ear that is surrounded the posterior groove of the superior antihelix crus and the posterior groove of the inferior antihelix crus. Clinically, many doctors use only that portion of the depression that is parallel with the groove is closest to the helix.

Functions: Calm the liver and extinguish wind; free the network vessels and relieve pain.

Indications: Hypertension, angioneurotic headache, facial paralysis.

UPPER EAR ROOT (MA-PS)

Location: The tip of the ear root that marks the superior attachment point of the ear.

Functions: Free the orifice and stanch bleeding.

Indications: Epistaxis.

ROOT OF EAR VAGUS (MA-PS)

Location: Corresponding to the helix root, at the juncture between the posterior ear and the mastoid process.

Functions: Course and disinhibit the liver and gallbladder; free the network vessels and relieve pain.

Indications: Cholecystitis, cholelithiasis, ascariasis of biliary tract, abdominal pain, diarrhea. This is also a supplementary point for treating arrhythmia.

LOWER EAR ROOT (MA-PS)

Location: At the lowermost rim of the root of the ear, where the ear cartilage is felt attached to the head.

Functions: Regulate the endocrine functions.

Indications: Low blood pressure, endocrine disturbance.

CHAPTER THREE

EAR DIAGNOSIS

THE THEORETICAL BASIS OF EAR DIAGNOSIS

The ear can theoretically be considered a complete, microcosmic representation that displays the physiological and pathological information of the entire body. Thus, when certain organs, tissues, or limbs are diseased, one can find positive reactions [i.e., showing the presence of a specific condition] in corresponding ear points. These positive reactions may present as lower electrical resistance, lower pain threshold, changes in color or appearance, desquamation, papular eruption, or congestion. Such positive reactions may be found even before a disease appears; they can disappear after treatment or remain forever. In addition, such reactions change over the course of a disease. In general, positive reactions not only identify the location and properties of a disorder, but also foretell the onset of diseases and their dynamic changes.

DIAGNOSTIC METHODS

The three most commonly used methods of diagnosis in ear acupuncture are (1) inspection, or visual observation, of changes in color and skin texture, (2) various palpation procedures, and (3) electrical detection of changes in the ear.

Ear Point Inspection Methods

Ear point inspection refers to visually observing pathological changes on the ear in terms of color, appearance, desquamation, papular eruption, and congestion. This method is generally used to diagnose acute and chronic diseases as well as to determine the location and properties of diseases.

APPLICATION

- Under natural light, pinch the auricle; look at the inside of the ear first, then the outside. Always observe the ear by looking from the upper part of the ear down to the lower part.

- When a possible positive reaction is found, use the index finger or middle finger to support the indicated area on the posterior surface and fully expose the position of the positive reaction to clearly observe its shape, size, color, hardness, and location.

- Observe both ears for comparison.

- If a cord or notch is found in the ear, the thumb, index finger, or a detection bar can be used to touch around it and determine its size, hardness, mobility, border, and tenderness.

- A detection bar or finger can be used to better expose areas around the helix root or antihelix crus.

CLASSIFICATION, PROPERTIES, AND CLINICAL SIGNIFICANCE OF POSITIVE REACTIONS

Color change

Red reaction: Bright red, light red, or dark red, which may be in spots or patches or have an irregular shape.

Bright red is seen in acute and painful disorders; light or dark red is often seen in recovery stages, chronic disorders, or protracted cases. For example, the area around Kidney (MA-SC) may present as a patchy, bright red in acute sprain of the lumbus; redness with desquamation can be found in the area around Uterus (MA-TF) in endometrial hyperplasia, cervicitis, and leukorrhea.

White reaction: White papular spots, patches with luster, or white spots edged by red.

A white reaction is mostly seen in chronic diseases such as chronic superficial gastritis. White spots edged by red are seen in chronic disorders with an acute onset, such as gastritis and rheumatic heart disease.

Gray reaction: Gray, light gray, or dark gray.

Gray is mostly seen in chronic diseases or various cancers.

Changes of Physical Shape

Projections: Projections can be as small as a sesame seed, as large as a green bean, or as hard as a soybean; they all project from the skin. Several projections may be linked together. Notch-like projections are mostly seen in hypertrophic arthritis; cord-like projections are seen in arthritis or myofibrositis; patch-like projections are seen in abdominal distention.

Pitting: Spot-like, patch-like, or linear pitting. Spot-like pitting is seen in tinnitus or astigmatism; patch-like pitting is seen in gastric and duodenal ulcers; linear pitting is seen in coronary heart disease, tinnitus, deafness, dental caries, and loss of teeth.

Projection with pitting: Seen with ametropia.

Rough, abnormally thickened, or wrinkled ear skin: Seen in dermal disorders.

Papular Eruption

Papular eruptions may be red, white, red-edged white, or dark gray eruptions, which are seen in acute or chronic organic disorders, or in allergic dermatitis. For example, a white, spot-like papular eruption is seen in cholelithiasis, bronchitis, or diarrhea; a flat, clustered eruption is seen in nodular prurigo.

Desquamation

With desquamation there is white chaff-like or scale-like skin sloughing. For example, desquamation occurring (a) in the triangular fossa indicates obstetric inflammation or leukorrhea; (b) at Esophagus (MA-IC6) and Cardiac (MA-IC7) indicates poor digestion; and (c) in the whole ear indicates seborrheic dermatitis.

Vascular Filling

The filling and shapes of blood vessels have various meanings. (a) Net-like filling indicates acute inflammation, such as pharyngitis, tonsillitis, or mastitis; (b) star-shaped vascular filling indicates ulcer; (c) circular or curved vascular filling indicates rheumatic heart disease; (d) vascular interruption indicates cardiac infarction.

CLASSIFICATION OF POSITIVE REACTIONS AND THEIR REGULARITY

Acute inflammation: Patchy, red congestion with seborrhea and luster, or in red with white edges in some cases.

Chronic organic diseases: Spot- or patch-like projection or pitting, white papular eruption without seborrhea and luster. Swelling can be found.

Various types of dermatitis: Chaff-like desquamation, papular eruption; rough, dark brown skin.

Cancer: Nodular projection or spot-like, dark gray millet.

Surgical scars: Linear or semi-lunar-shaped marks that are white or dark grey.

The principles for ear point inspection can be summarized as follows: a red color indicates an acute condition while a white color with pitting or projection indicates a chronic condition. Desquamation indicates inflammation and squamous tuberculous disorders on the skin. Linear or semi-lunar-shaped white or dim gray color indicates surgical scarring; nodular projections that are dark gray indicate cancer.

PRIMARY POINTS FOR ATTENTION

- Practitioners should be familiar with the location and distribution pattern of points, and should thoroughly understand the theories of TCM and Western medicine.

- Inspection should be done in natural lighting.

- The ear should not be washed before inspection in order to avoid altering any positive reactions. If necessary, use a dry cotton ball to clean the ear, wiping in one direction only, but do not scrub.

- Visual inspection should be done in combination with palpation.

- Pseudo-positive reactions, such as may occur with nevus or frostbite, should be ruled out. If points visually appear to present a positive reaction, yet pressure with a detection bar registers no sensation of soreness, numbness, or pain, the appearance should be considered a pseudo-positive reaction.

- Individual constitution, race, skin color, sex, age, and the season should be taken into account during inspection.

- Pattern identification according to the theory of bowels and viscera should be applied when a positive reaction is found.

Ear Point Palpation Methods

Palpation should be performed on the basis of inspection. It can be done with the fingers, a detection bar, or an electrical detector.

PALPATION OF SENSITIVE SPOTS

Palpating sensitive spots is useful in diagnosing the location and properties of acute diseases and painful disorders. The sensitive spots should also be used for treatment. Severity of pain may be divided into degrees for ease of comparison; the severity of pain is determined by the patient's reaction when the points are pressed. In general, the stronger the pain, the more severe the disease.

EXTERNAL ELEMENT PRESSING

External element pressing is useful in diagnosing the location and properties of chronic diseases during a patient's follow-up visits, as well as for health screening. The detection should be done in an orderly manner, such as according to anatomical areas (as described below).

Projections, pitting, nodes, cords, hyperplasia of cartilage, and edema should be further inspected with this method.

RUBBING

Rubbing is suitable for diagnosing various chronic and organic diseases. With the thumb and index finger, palpate deeply into the auricular tissues to find subdermal pathological changes.

Hyperplasia of cartilage, nodes, projections, and cords, and the size, hardness, and tenderness of each, can be identified with touching.

ELECTRICAL DETECTION

A variety of electrical detection devices can be used to determine electrical resistance at ear points. Because information about the body collects at the ear, when an organ or part of the body is ailing, the electrical resistance at corresponding ear points will change significantly.

Order of Examination

In performing ear diagnosis, the convention is to work through the different areas of the ear in the following sequences.

According to anatomical areas: (1) Triangular fossa, (2) concha, (3) helix root, (4) antitragus, (5) intertragic notch, (6) tragus, (7) lobe, (8) antihelix, (9) superior crus of antihelix, (10) inferior crus of antihelix, (11) scaphoid fossa, (12) helix, (13) posterior surface of ear.

According to physiological systems: (1) blood pressure, (2) obstetric and reproductive system, (3) urinary system, (4) liver and gallbladder, (5) stomach and intestines, (6) cardiovascular and respiratory system, (7) nervous system, (8) face and eye, nose, mouth, tongue, and throat, and (9) trunk and extremities.

Positive Reaction

Beeps will be heard when an electric detector is located at areas where electrical resistance is lower. Positive reactions are divided into three degrees:

Mild positive reaction (±)
> The beeps occur slowly, with low sound, low tone, and low frequency; there is no specific pain at the tested area.

Positive reaction (+)
> Beeps occur quickly with loud sound, low tone, and unchanging frequency; there is tenderness at the tested area.

Strong positive reaction (++)
> Beeps occur quickly with loud sound and the tone changes
> from low to high; there is pricking pain at the tested area.

AURICULAR DIAGNOSIS IN COMMONLY SEEN DISORDERS

Internal Diseases

ACUTE GASTRITIS

Inspection: Patchy redness with luster at Stomach (MA-IC).
Palpation: Tenderness at Stomach (MA-IC).
Electrical Detection: Positive reaction (+) at Stomach (MA-IC).

CHRONIC GASTRITIS

Superficial Gastritis

Inspection: White patchy projection without clear edges at Stomach (MA-IC).
Palpation: Patch-like projection, hard and cord-like, at Stomach (MA-IC).
Electrical Detection: Positive reaction (+) at Stomach (MA-IC).

Hypertrophic Gastritis

Inspection: Large projection with clearly defined edges at Stomach (MA-IC).
Palpation: Large projection with hardness at Stomach (MA-IC).
Electrical Detection: Positive reaction (+) at Stomach (MA-IC).

Atrophic Gastritis

Inspection: Flat or pitting with wrinkles in red alternating with white at Stomach (MA-IC).
Palpation: Tenderness at Stomach (MA-IC).
Electrical Detection: Positive reaction (+) at Stomach (MA-IC).

CHRONIC GASTRITIS WITH ACUTE ATTACK

Inspection: Patch-like white projection alternating with spotty red with luster.
Palpation: Tenderness at Stomach (MA-IC).
Electrical Detection: Positive to strong positive reaction (+ to ++).

GASTRIC ULCER

Active Phase

> **Inspection:** Spot- or patch-like congestion with clearly defined edges and luster, sometimes with a millet-like pitting in the middle at Stomach (MA-IC).
>
> **Palpation:** Pitting caused by touching, tenderness at Stomach (MA-IC).
>
> **Electrical Detection:** Positive reaction (+) at Stomach (MA-IC).

Resting Phase

> **Inspection:** Spot- or patch-like pitting in dark purple at Stomach (MA-IC).
>
> **Palpation:** Pitting caused by touching at Stomach (MA-IC).
>
> **Electrical Detection:** Mild positive reaction (±) at Stomach (MA-IC).

Recovery Phase

> **Inspection:** Spot- or patch-like projection with clearly defined edges at Stomach (MA-IC).
>
> **Palpation:** Cord-like projection at Stomach (MA-IC).
>
> **Electrical Detection:** Mild positive reaction (±) at Stomach (MA-IC).

DUODENAL ULCER

Active Phase

> **Inspection:** Millet-like pitting in red, with clearly defined edges at Duodenum (MA-SC1); a defect occurring at the lateral third of the superior border of helix root; vascular filling radiating to Pancreas/Gallbladder (MA-SC6).
>
> **Palpation:** Severe tenderness at Duodenum (MA-SC1).
>
> **Electrical Detection:** Strong positive reaction (++) at Duodenum (MA-SC1).

Resting Phase

> **Inspection:** Millet-like pitting in dark purple with clearly defined edges at Duodenum (MA-SC1), capillary filling radiating to superior border of helix root.
>
> **Palpation:** Tenderness at Duodenum (MA-SC1).
>
> **Electrical Detection:** Positive reaction (+) at Duodenum (MA-SC1).

Recovery Phase

Inspection: Millet-like pitting in dark brown, with clearly defined edges at Duodenum (MA-SC1), capillary filling radiating to the superior border of helix root.

Palpation: Cord-like projection without tenderness at Duodenum (MA-SC1).

Electrical Detection: Mild positive reaction (±) at Duodenum (MA-SC1).

DUODENAL BULBAR INFLAMMATION

Inspection: Patch-like redness with undefined edges at Duodenum (MA-SC1).

Palpation: Mild pitting at Duodenum (MA-SC1).

Electrical Detection: Positive reaction (+) at Duodenum (MA-SC1)

ACUTE ENTERITIS

Inspection: Patch-like vascular filling in red with luster and seborrhea at Large Intestine (MA-SC4). Sometimes papular eruptions can be found around the area.

Palpation: Flat or pitting, tenderness at Large Intestine (MA-SC4).

Electrical Detection: Positive reaction (+) at Large Intestine (MA-SC4).

CHRONIC DIARRHEA

Inspection: Patch-like pitting in dark red with seborrhea at Large Intestine (MA-SC4).

Palpation: Patch-like pitting, tenderness at Large Intestine (MA-SC4).

Electrical Detection: Positive reaction (+) at Large Intestine (MA-SC4).

Allergic colitis is indicated if a positive reaction is found at Wind Stream (MA-SF) and Endocrine (MA-IC3) together with Large Intestine (MA-SC4).

CONSTIPATION

Inspection: Patch- or cord-like projection with chaff-like desquamation at Large Intestine (MA-SC4).

Palpation: Cord-like, hard projection at Large Intestine (MA-SC4).

Electrical Detection: Mild positive reaction (±) at Large Intestine (MA-SC4).

INTESTINAL FUNCTIONAL DISTURBANCE

Inspection: White, patch-like projection at Small Intestine (MA-SC2). Flatness or red or dark purple pitting at Large Intestine (MA-SC4).

Palpation: Patch-like projection at Small Intestine (MA-SC2), flatness or pitting at Large Intestine (MA-SC4) without tenderness.

Electrical Detection: Positive reaction (+) at Large Intestine (MA-SC4), Small Intestine (MA-SC2), Wind Stream (MA-SF), Spleen (MA-IC) and Subcortex (MA-AT1).

INFANTILE MALNUTRITION

Electrical Detection: Positive reaction (+) at Spleen (MA-IC), Endocrine (MA-IC3) and Subcortex (MA-AT1).

ACUTE HEPATITIS

Inspection: Spot- or patch-like redness with luster at Liver (MA-SC5).

Palpation: Pitting in red after pressing, tenderness at Liver (MA-SC5).

Electrical Detection: Positive reaction (+) at Liver (MA-SC5).

CHRONIC HEPATITIS

Inspection: White, patch-like projection at Liver (MA-SC5).
Palpation: Patch-like projection, tenderness at Liver (MA-SC5).
Electrical Detection: Positive reaction (+) at Liver (MA-SC5).

CIRRHOSIS OF THE LIVER

Inspection: Dark color at Liver (MA-SC5); patch-like projection at Spleen (MA-IC).

Palpation: No tenderness at Liver (MA-SC5) but cord-like projection at Spleen (MA-IC) and Esophagus (MA-IC6).

Electrical Detection: Positive reaction (+) can be found at Subcortex (MA-AT1), Endocrine (MA-IC3), Spleen (MA-IC), Esophagus (MA-IC6), and Liver (MA-SC5).

HEPATOMEGALY

Inspection: White projection with clearly defined edges at Liver (MA-SC5).

Palpation: Cord-like projection at Liver (MA-SC5).
Electrical Detection: Mild positive reaction (±) at Liver (MA- SC5).

ACUTE CHOLECYSTITIS

Inspection: Patch-like redness with luster at Pancreas/Gallbladder (MA- SC6).

Palpation: Obvious tenderness at Gallbladder (MA-SC6).

Electrical Detection: Positive reaction (+) at Pancreas/Gallbladder (MA-SC6).

CHRONIC CHOLECYSTITIS

Inspection: White, patch- or cord-like projection at Pancreas/Gallbladder (MA-SC6).

Palpation: Hard, patch- or cord-like projection at Pancreas/Gallbladder (MA-SC6), tenderness.

Electrical Detection: Mild positive reaction (±) at Pancreas/Gallbladder (MA-SC6).

CHOLELITHIASIS

Inspection: One or several papular eruptions or nodes at Liver of Posterior Surface (MA-PS);[5] white, patch-like projection at Pancreas/Gallbladder (MA-SC6).

Palpation: Round nodes or cords at Pancreas/Gallbladder (MA-SC6) and Liver of Posterior Surface (MA-PS).

Electrical Detection: Positive to strong positive reaction (+ to ++) at Pancreas/Gallbladder (MA-SC6) and Liver of Posterior Surface (MA-PS).

CHRONIC CHOLANGITIS

Inspection: Patch-like redness or dark purple pitting or capillary filling at Pancreas/Gallbladder (MA-SC6) and Duodenum (MA-SC1).

Palpation: Pitting, cord- or patch-like projection, tenderness at Pancreas/Gallbladder (MA-SC6).

Electrical Detection: Positive to strong positive reaction (+ to ++) at Pancreas/Gallbladder (MA-SC6).

SPLENOMEGALY

Inspection: Dark red projection at Spleen (MA-IC) on the left ear.

Palpation: Cord-like projection, pitting by pressing in area above Spleen (MA-IC).

Electrical Detection: Positive reaction (+) at Spleen (MA-IC).

---

[5] *Editor's Note:* Though all the posterior surface areas are named for zang organs, they retain their fu organ correspondences for treatment purposes where necessary.

COMMON COLD

> **Electrical Detection:** Positive reaction (+) at Lung (MA-IC1),
> Pharynx and Larynx (MA-T3), Internal Nose (MA-T) and
> Bronchii/Trachea (MA-IC2).

CHRONIC BRONCHITIS

> **Inspection:** White, patch-like projection at Bronchii/Trachea
> (MA-IC2), white papular eruptions without luster in some
> cases.
> **Palpation:** Patch- or cord-like projection at Bronchii/Trachea
> (MA-IC2), no obvious tenderness.
> **Electrical Detection:** Positive reaction (+) at Bronchii/Trachea
> (MA-IC2).

BRONCHIAL ASTHMA

> **Inspection:** White, flat projection at Bronchii/Trachea (MA-IC2);
> white rash without luster in same area in some cases.
> **Palpation:** Flat or linear projection at Bron-
> chii/Trachea (MA-IC2), slightly tender.
> **Electrical Detection:** Positive reaction (+) at Bronchii/Trachea
> (MA-IC2), Lung (MA-IC1), Wind Stream (MA-SF), Endo-
> crine (MA- IC3), and Apex of Antitragus (MA-AT).

BRONCHIECTASIS

> **Inspection:** Dark red cord-like projection, without luster, at
> Lung (MA-IC1) and Trachea (MA-IC2); capillary filling can
> be found over Lung (MA-IC1).
> **Palpation:** Several cord-like projections at Lung (MA-IC1) and
> Trachea (MA-IC2).
> **Electrical Detection:** Positive reaction (+) at Bronchii/Trachea
> (MA-IC2).

PULMONARY TUBERCULOSIS

Active Phase

> **Inspection:** Red, patch-like, papular eruptions with luster at
> Lung (MA-IC1).
> **Palpation:** Bumpiness at Lung (MA-IC1).
> **Electrical Detection:** Strong positive reaction (++) at area around
> Lung (MA-IC1).

Calcification Phase

> **Inspection:** One or several needlepoint pitting areas alternating
> with dark gray spots or patch-like eruptions, with clearly de-
> fined edges, in the area around Lung (MA-IC1).

Palpation: Cord-like projection or node at Lung (MA-IC1).
Electrical Detection: Positive reaction (+) at Lung (MA-IC1).

HYPERTENSION

Inspection: Flatness (-) or projection (+) at Blood Pressure Raising Point (*Shēng Yā Diǎn,* at the lower rim of the root of the ear, in the Tooth area).

Electrical Detection: Strong positive reaction (++) at Blood Pressure Lowering Point (*Jiàng Yā Diǎn,* in the Superior Triangular Fossa).

CORONARY HEART DISEASE

Palpation is mainly performed in the left ear for this disease.

Palpation: Edema with pitting at Heart (MA-IC); undulating edema when pressing the area around Heart (MA-IC); cord- or patch-like projection above or below Heart (MA-IC); stabbing pain at Heart (MA-IC); thin, easily broken skin at Heart (MA-IC).

Electrical Detection: Positive to strong positive reaction (+ to ++) at Heart (MA-IC).

PAROXYSMAL TACHYCARDIA

Palpation: Cord- or patch-like projection at the inferior quarter of the border of Heart (MA-IC), tenderness.

Electrical Detection: Positive reaction (+) at Heart (MA-IC), Heart of Posterior Surface (MA-PS), and Subcortex (MA-AT1).

BRADYCARDIA

Inspection: Normal physiological pitting disappears at Heart (MA-IC), which presents flat or with slight bulges.
Palpation: Bumpiness at Heart (MA-IC).
Electrical Detection: Positive reaction (+) at Heart (MA-IC).

ATRIOVENTRICULAR BLOCK

Inspection: Brown, needlepoint-sized, papular eruptions at Heart (MA-IC) are seen in incomplete block of bundle branch.

PREMATURE HEARTBEAT

Palpation: Ring-like, pitting edema at Heart (MA-IC).
Electrical Detection: Positive reaction (+) at Heart (MA-IC) and Subcortex (MA-AT1).

RHEUMATIC HEART DISEASE

Inspection: Bumpy change of an irregular shape and dark color and capillary filling with clear edge at Heart (MA-IC) involving the inferior border of the helix root and Spleen (MA-IC).

Palpation: Irregular-shaped, bumpy change at Heart (MA-IC), stabbing pain.

Electrical Detection: Strong positive reaction (++) at Heart (MA-IC).

ENLARGEMENT OF HEART

Inspection: Wrinkled, red, round, or ellipsoid 0.5 x 0.5 cm shape, near Heart (MA-IC).

Palpation: Unevenness at Heart (MA-IC).

Electrical Detection: Positive reaction (+) at Heart (MA-IC).

FRONTAL HEADACHE

Inspection: Projection at Forehead (MA-AT).

Palpation: Round, cord- or patch-like projection, soft in quality at Forehead (MA-AT).

Electrical Detection: Positive reaction (+) at Forehead (MA-AT).

MIGRAINE HEADACHE

Inspection: Patch-like projection at Temple (MA-AT).

Palpation: Tenderness at Temple (MA-AT).

Electrical Detection: Positive reaction (+) at Temple (MA-AT).

OCCIPITAL HEADACHE

Inspection: Patch-like projection at Occiput (MA-AT).

Palpation: Projection, soft in quality, at Occiput (MA-AT).

Electrical Detection: Positive reaction (+) at Occiput (MA-AT).

HEADACHE OCCURRING IN THE WHOLE HEAD

Inspection: Patch-like projection on lateral surface of antitragus, Occiput (MA-AT), Temple (MA-AT), and Forehead (MA-AT).

Palpation: Unevenness on lateral surface of antitragus, or cord-like projection.

DIZZINESS

Inspection: Red, cord- or patch-like pitting with luster at Occiput (MA-AT).

Palpation: Pitting at Occiput (MA-AT).

Electrical Detection: Positive reaction (+) at Occiput (MA-AT).

NEUROSIS

Inspection: Irregular-shaped projection between Cervical Vertebrae (MA-AH8) and Occiput (MA-AT).

Palpation: Hardened cord- or patch-like thickening of cartilage that can be felt by pinching in the area between Cervical Vertebrae (MA-AH8) and Occiput (MA-AT).

Electrical Detection: Positive to strong positive reaction (+ to ++) at Heart (MA-IC), Subcortex (MA-AT1) and in the area between Cervical Vertebrae (MA-AH8) and Occiput (MA-AT).

AUTONOMIC NERVOUS SYSTEM FUNCTIONAL DISTURBANCE

Electrical Detection: Positive reaction (+) at Sympathetic (MA-AH7), Heart (MA-IC), Kidney (MA-SC), Occiput (MA-AT), Forehead (MA-AT), and Subcortex (MA-AT1).

TRIGEMINAL NEURALGIA

Palpation: Severe tenderness at Jaw (MA-L), Tongue (MA-L), Eye (MA-L1), and Cheek (MA-L); pain threshold in ear of the affected side is obviously lower than in the healthy side.

Electrical Detection: Positive reaction (+) at Cheek (MA-L), Mouth (MA-IC5), and Triple Burner (MA-IC4).

CHRONIC NEPHRITIS

Inspection: White, patch-like projection or papular eruption, with luster at Kidney (MA-SC)

Palpation: Stabbing pain at Kidney (MA-SC), Endocrine (MA-IC3), Wind Stream (MA-SF), and Kidney of Posterior Surface (MA-PS); pitting edema at Kidney (MA-SC).

Electrical Detection: Positive reaction (+) at Kidney (MA-SC), Endocrine (MA-IC3), Wind Stream (MA-SF) and Kidney of Posterior Surface (MA-PS).

CHRONIC PYELONEPHRITIS

Palpation: Tenderness at Kidney (MA-SC) and Urethra (MA-H3); cord-like projection at Urethra (MA-H3).

Electrical Detection: Positive reaction (+) at Kidney (MA-SC) and Urethra (MA-H3).

CHRONIC CYSTITIS

Palpation: Tenderness at Bladder (MA-SC8) and Urethra (MA-H3); cord-like projection at Urethra (MA-H3).

Electrical Detection: Mild positive reaction (±) at Bladder (MA-SC8) and Urethra (MA-H3).

DIABETES

Inspection: White swelling at Pancreas/Gallbladder (MA-SC6).

Palpation: Pitting edema at Pancreas/Gallbladder (MA-SC6). In general, it is found that the more severe the edema, the higher the blood sugar.

Electrical Detection: Strong positive reaction (++) at Pancreas/Gallbladder (MA-SC6) and Endocrine (MA-IC3).

CHRONIC PROSTATITIS

Palpation: Tenderness at Prostate/Angle of Superior Concha (MA-SC) and Urethra (MA-H3).

Electrical Detection: Positive reaction (+) at Prostate/Angle of Superior Concha (MA-SC) and Urethra (MA-H3).

PROSTATIC HYPERTROPHY

Inspection: Dull and bulging change of Prostate/Angle of Superior Concha.

Palpation: Hardened projection at Prostate/Angle of Superior Concha (MA-SC); cord-like projection at Urethra (MA-H3).

Electrical Detection: Positive reaction (+) at Urethra (MA-H3) and Prostate/Angle of Superior Concha (MA-SC).

URINARY TRACT INFECTION

Palpation: Tenderness at Urethra (MA-H3), Bladder (MA-SC8) and Prostate/Angle of Superior Concha (MA-SC); cord-like projection at Urethra (MA-H3).

Electrical Detection: Positive reaction (+) at Urethra (MA-H3), Bladder (MA-SC8), and Prostate/Angle of Superior Concha (MA-SC).

External diseases

ACUTE TRAUMATIC INJURY OF JOINT AND SOFT TISSUE

Inspection: Patchy red with swelling at corresponding points.

Palpation: Pitting edema with tenderness at the corresponding points.

Electrical Detection: Positive to strong positive reaction (+ to ++) at corresponding points (e.g., shoulder disorder – shoulder point; heel disorder – heel point).

OLD TRAUMATIC INJURY OF JOINT AND SOFT TISSUE

Inspection: Projections at the corresponding points.

Palpation: Cord- or patch-like projections at the corresponding points.
Electrical Detection: Mild positive to positive reaction (± to +) at the corresponding points.

ACUTE ARTHRITIS

Inspection: Patchy redness, bright-red capillary filling at the corresponding points.
Palpation: Red patch or spotty pitting edema, severe tenderness at the corresponding points.
Electrical Detection: Positive to strong positive reaction (+ to ++) at the corresponding points.

CHRONIC ARTHRITIS

Inspection: White, spotty projections at the corresponding points.
Palpation: Unevenness at the surface of the corresponding points; cord-like projections.
Electrical Detection: Positive reaction (+) at the corresponding points.

LUMBAR MUSCLE STRAIN

Inspection: For chronic strain, irregularly shaped white projections are seen at Lumbosacrat Vertebrae (MA-AH); for acute strain, red projections with luster and capillary filling is seen.
Palpation: Deformation at Lumbosacral Vertebrae (MA-AH).
Electrical Detection: Strong positive reaction (++) at Lumbosacral Vertebrae (MA-AH).

HYPERPLASIA OF LUMBAR VERTEBRAE

Inspection: Nodule or bead-like projection at Lumbosacral Vertebrae (MA-AH).
Palpation: Cord-like projection at Lumbar Vertebrae (MA-AH).
Electrical Detection: Positive reaction (+) at Lumbosacral Vertebrae (MA-AH).

MYOFIBROSITIS OF SHOULDER AND BACK

Inspection: White projection at lateral rim of antitragus.
Palpation: Hyperplasia and deformation of cartilage, hard in quality.
Electrical Detection: Positive reaction (+) at the corresponding area in the auricle.

HYPERPLASIA OF CALCANEUS

Palpation: Tenderness, cord-like projections at Heel (MA-AH1).

Electrical Detection: Positive reaction (+) at Heel (MA-AH1).

SPASM OF CALF

Electrical Detection: Positive reaction (+) at the corresponding point in auricle.

SCIATICA

Electrical Detection: Positive reaction (+) at Hip (MA-AH4), Buttocks (MA-AH5), Knee (MA-AH3), Ankle (MA-AH2), Heel (MA-AH1), and Toe (MA-AH).

SPONDYLOPATHY

Inspection: Nodule or bead-like deformation at Cervical Vertebrae (MA-AH8).
Palpation: Hyperplasia of cartilage, cord-like projection at Cervical Vertebrae (MA-AH8).
Electrical Detection: Mild positive to positive reaction (± to +) at Cervical Vertebrae (MA-AH8).

CHRONIC APPENDICITIS

Inspection: White patch-like projection at Appendix (MA-SC3).
Palpation: Cord-like projection at Appendix (MA-SC3).
Electrical Detection: Mild positive reaction (±) at Appendix (MA-SC3).

HEMORRHOID

Inspection: Uneven on the surface around Anus (MA-H5), spot- or patch-like redness or capillary filling at Anus (MA-H5) is seen in thrombosed external hemorrhoid.
Palpation: Cord-like projection at Anus (MA-H5) in external hemorrhoid.
Electrical Detection: Mild positive reaction (±) at Anus (MA-H5) is seen in thrombosed external hemorrhoid.

ANAL FISSURE

Inspection: Red nodular or serrated change at Anus (MA-H5)
Palpation: Nodular or cord-like projection at Anus (MA-H5).
Electrical Detection: Positive reaction (+) at Anus (MA-H5).

SEXUAL HYPOFUNCTION

Electrical Detection: Positive reaction (+) at Internal Reproductive Organs (MA-TF), Pelvis (MA-TF), Prostate/Angle of Superior Concha (MA-SC), Urethra (MA-H3), Testicle (MA-AT), Kidney (MA-SC), and Endocrine (MA-IC3).

Gynecological and Obstetric Diseases

PELVIC INFLAMMATION

Inspection: Patch-like projection and spot-like redness at Pelvis (MA-TF).

Palpation: Cord-like projection at Pelvis (MA-TF).

Electrical Detection: Positive reaction (+) at Pelvis (MA-TF).

ADNEXITIS

Inspection: Cord- or patch-like projection and spot-like redness at Adnexa (Fù Jiàng)[6] (corresponding to the adnexa uteri), located in the upper 1/3 portion of Internal Reproductive Organs (MA-TF).

Palpation: Cord- or patch-like projection at Fù Jiàng, the corresponding point of adnexa uteri in the ear. Inflammation may be occurring in both adnexa (ovaries) if the changes are found in both ears.

Electrical Detection: Positive reaction (+) at Fù Jiàng.

CERVICITIS

Inspection: Patch-like pitting, redness, seborrhea, desquamation, and papular eruption at Cervix (MA-TF, Gōng Jǐng).[7]

Palpation: Skin at Cervix (MA-TF, Gōng Jǐng) becomes thinner, is easily broken, or has spot-like capillary filling and tenderness.

Electrical Detection: Positive reaction (+) at Cervix (MA-TF).

MENSTRUAL DISORDERS

Profuse, Advanced Menstruation

Inspection: Redness with luster edged by swelling in white at Uterus (MA-TF).

Palpation: Pitting edema at Uterus (Zǐ Gōng, MA-TF).[8]

Electrical Detection: Positive to strong positive reaction (+ to ++) at Uterus (MA-TF).

Scant, Delayed Menstruation

Inspection: Flat change at triangular fossa.

---

[6] Fù Jiàng refers generally to the female reproductive organs and specifically can refer to the ovaries and fallopian tubes.

[7] Cervix (MA-TF) is located in the lower 1/3 portion of Internal Reproductive Organs (MA-TF).

[8] Uterus (MA-TF) is located in the middle 1/3 portion of Internal Reproductuve Organs (MA-TF)

Palpation: Hardened, patch- or cord-like projection at Uterus (MA-TF).

Electrical Detection: Positive reaction (+) at Uterus (MA-TF).

DYSFUNCTIONAL UTERINE BLEEDING

Inspection: White, patch-like swelling at triangular fossa.

Palpation: Pitting edema involving triangular fossa.

Electrical Detection: Strong positive reaction (++) at Uterus (MA-TF); mild positive to positive reaction (± to +) at Liver (MA-SC5), Spleen (MA-IC), and Kidney (MA-SC).

HYSTEROMYOMA

Palpation: Cord-like hyperplasia or node at Uterus (MA-TF); cord-like projection at Internal Reproductive Organs (MA-TF) and Endocrine (MA-IC3).

Electrical Detection: Positive reaction (+) at Uterus (*Zĭ Gōng*, MA-TF).

LEUKORRHEA

Inspection: Redness, seborrhea, and desquamation or spot-like papular eruption at triangular fossa.

Palpation: Red pitting at triangular fossa.

Electrical Detection: Positive reaction (+) at triangular fossa.

Dermal Diseases

ACUTE URTICARIA

Inspection: Redness at Wind Stream (MA-SF).

Palpation: Red, pitting edema at Wind Stream (MA-SF).

Electrical Detection: Positive to strong positive reaction (+ to ++) at Wind Stream (MA-SF).

CHRONIC URTICARIA

Inspection: Redness at Wind Stream (MA-SF), bran-like desquamation at Lung (MA-IC1).

Palpation: White, pitting edema at Wind Stream (MA-SF).

Electrical Detection: Positive reaction (+) at Wind Stream (MA-SF).

NEURODERMATITIS

Inspection: Bran-like desquamation at Lung (MA-IC1); rough, dark brown change on the surface of this area.

Palpation: Tenderness at Lung (MA-IC1).

Electrical Detection: Mild positive reaction (±) at Lung (MA-IC1).

SEBORRHEIC DERMATITIS

Inspection: Seborrheic desquamation in the whole auricle; occasionally, patch-like glossy redness can be found.

Electrical Detection: Positive reaction (+) at Lung (MA-IC1) and Endocrine (MA-IC3).

CUTANEOUS PRURITUS

Inspection: Dry skin and desquamation without luster in the whole auricle, particularly at Lung (MA-IC1) and Wind Stream (MA-SF).

Electrical Detection: Positive reaction (+) at Lung (MA-IC1) and Wind Stream (MA-SF).

Disorders of the Eye, Nose, Ear, Mouth, and Throat

CHRONIC PHARYNGITIS

Inspection: Edema at Mouth (MA-IC5) and Bronchii/Trachea (MA-IC2).

Palpation: Spot-like pitting at Bronchii/Trachea (MA-IC2).

Electrical Detection: Positive reaction (+) at Pharynx and Larynx (MA-T3), Bronchii/Trachea (MA-IC2), and Mouth (MA-IC5).

CHRONIC TONSILLITIS

Inspection: Dark purple or red patch-like projection at Tonsil (MA-L).

Palpation: Cord-like projection at Tonsil (MA-L).

Electrical Detection: Positive reaction (+) at Mouth (MA-IC5), Pharynx and Larynx (MA-T3), and Tonsil (MA-L).

CHRONIC RHINITIS

Inspection: No deformation or color change at Internal Nose (MA-T).

Electrical Detection: Positive reaction (+) at Internal Nose (MA-T).

ALLERGIC RHINITIS

Inspection: White, patch-like projection resembling edema at Internal Nose (MA-T).

Palpation: Pitting edema at Internal Nose (MA-T) and Wind Stream (MA-SF).

Electrical Detection: Positive reaction (+) at Internal Nose (MA-T) and Wind Stream (MA-SF).

NASOSINUSITIS

Inspection: Patch-like projection at Internal Nose (MA-T), irregular-shaped projection at Forehead (MA-AT).

Palpation: Hardened projection at Internal Nose (MA-T).

Electrical Detection: Positive reaction (+) at Internal Nose (MA-T), Lung (MA-IC1), and Forehead (MA-AT).

GINGIVAL BLEEDING

Inspection: Patch-like projection and edema at Jaw (MA-L) and Mouth (MA-IC5) involving Bronchii/Trachea (MA-IC2).

Palpation: Pitting edema at Bronchii/Trachea (MA-IC2) and Mouth (MA-IC5); soft projection at Jaw (MA-L).

Electrical Detection: Positive reaction (+) at Mouth (MA-IC5) and Jaw (MA-L).

GINGIVITIS

Inspection: Patch-like projection and edema at Mouth (MA-IC5) and Jaw (MA-L).

Palpation: Soft, patch- or cord-like projection at Mouth (MA-IC5) and Jaw (MA-L).

Electrical Detection: Positive reaction (+) at Mouth (MA-IC5) and Jaw (MA-L).

DENTAL CARIES

Inspection: Spot-like or thready pitting with wrinkled skin at Jaw (MA-L).

Palpation: Pitting when Jaw (MA-L) is pressed.

Electrical Detection: Positive reaction (+) at Jaw (MA-L).

SORES IN MOUTH

Inspection: Projection at Mouth (MA-IC5) and Tongue (MA-L).

Palpation: Patch- or cord-like projection at Mouth (MA-IC5) and Tongue (MA-L).

Electrical Detection: Positive reaction (+) at ear lobe.

MYOPIA

Inspection: Patch-like projection at posterior of intertragic notch.

Palpation: Irregular, soft projection in posterior of intertragic notch.

Electrical Detection: Positive reaction (+) in posterior of intertragic notch and Eye (MA-L1).

ASTIGMATISM

> **Inspection:** Spot-like or irregular pitting between posterior of the intertragic notch and Forehead (MA-AT).
>
> **Palpation:** Pitting between posterior of intertragic notch and Forehead (MA-AT).
>
> **Electrical Detection:** Positive reaction (+) at Forehead (MA-AT), Eye (MA-L1), and posterior of intertragic notch.

CHAPTER FOUR

THERAPEUTIC METHODS

Once a diagnosis is made, ear acupuncturists have a wide range of therapeutic methods to apply on ear points. This chapter explains in detail the procedures used for seed acupressure, needling ear points, implanting needles, electroacupuncture, plum-blossom needling, bloodletting, medicine injection, moxibustion, massage, medicinal plasters, and magnet therapy. It also introduces several treatment methods that have been used in China yet which are not likely to be used widely in other countries.

SEED ACUPRESSURE

In seed acupressure (which is sometimes called "pill acupressure" or "bead acupressure"), plant seeds, medicinal pills, or magnetic beads are affixed to ear points with adhesive strips as an alternative to using needles. This method is simple to use, widely applicable, and has a superior effect because it affords continuous stimulation. It is also safe, free of side effects, and economical. Its popularity in the clinic has grown steadily, especially in treating older adults and infants.

Materials

SEEDS, PILLS AND OTHER MATERIAL FOR PRESSING

Any seed or pill having a smooth surface of a suitable size and hardness can be used for seed acupressure, including vaccaria seed (*wáng bù liú xíng zǐ*), radish seed (*lái fú zǐ*), white mustard seed (*bái jiè zǐ*), cuscuta seed (*tù sī zǐ*), rapeseed (*yóu cài zǐ*), fetid cassia seed (*jué míng zǐ*), spiny jujuba kernel (*suān zǎo rén*), alpinia seed (*yì zhì rén*), rice bean (*chì xiǎo dòu*), and mung bean (*lù dòu*). Choose mature seeds (or beans) with a diameter of

1.0–1.5mm. Boil in water for two minutes, then dry for use. Magnetic beads and borneol are also commonly used for this treatment method. Certain medicinal pills can also be used, such as Six Spirits Pill (*Lìu Shén Wán*) and Sore Throat Pill (*Hóu Zhèng Wán*). Of all these materials, vaccaria seeds and magnetic beads are the most commonly used.

EQUIPMENT

Adhesive strips, cut into pieces of approximately 14mm x 14mm; 75% alcohol; 2.5% iodine tincture; sterilized, dry cotton balls; a surgical knife; and tweezers.

Points for Attention

- Do not allow adhesive strips to become wet, as this may cause skin infection. For those who have an allergic reaction to adhesive strips and present with red papular eruptions and itching in the ear, perform bloodletting at Ear Apex (MA-H6) or give allergy medications.

- Use fewer ear points in summer. The treatment course should also be shorter to avoid skin infection in the ear.

- Do not use ear acupressure on patients with dermal disorders such as frostbite and eczema.

- If pain occurs in the treated ear during sleep, the adhesive strip with seeds can be loosened or even taken off according to the patient's wishes.

- Manipulate the seeds gently for infants and pregnant women.

- Patients with hypertension, coronary heart disease, and arteriosclerosis should have adequate rest before treatments. Careful observation should be done after treating such patients to prevent accidents.

Procedure

IDENTIFICATION OF SENSITIVE POINTS

First, determine the prescription according to ear diagnosis; next, identify sensitive spots in selected point areas according to inspection, tenderness, and electrical detection.

STERILIZATION OF AREA TO BE TREATED

Sterilize the area to be treated or, if necessary, the whole ear with 75% alcohol.

APPLYING THE BANDAGE

Place the seed in the center of a small piece of adhesive strip. Hold the ear gently using the thumb, middle, and index fingers, then affix the prepared bandage on the selected ear point with tweezers. Press the seed firmly into place.

ACUPRESSURE

Apply gradually increasing pressure to the seeds until reaching the patient's level of tolerance. Continue pressing until heat, distention, or a rush of blood is felt in the auricle. In general, use mild stimulation for weaker patients, older adults, pregnant women, and infants; use stronger pressure for acute, febrile, or painful disorders. For painful disorders, maintain pressure until the pain is relieved.

TREATMENT COURSE

In general, treatment is performed in only one ear at three to five points, changing ears every five to seven days. Both ears can be treated when necessary.

Following treatment by a practitioner, the patient should press the seeds three to five times each day, holding the pressure for two to three minutes each time.

Commonly Used Seeds for Acupressure

VACCARIA SEED

The most commonly used seed for acupressure is vaccaria seed with a diameter of 2mm. Most disorders can be treated with vaccaria seed acupressure.

MUNG BEAN

Mung beans clear heat and resolve toxins and summerheat; they are used to treat diseases of a hot nature. Due to their large size, mung beans should be cut in half; apply the smooth surface to the ear point.

FETID CASSIA SEED

Cassia seeds clear heat and brighten the eyes, moisten the intestine and free the stool; thus, cassia seed acupressure is used to treat disorders of the eyes and head as well as for constipation.

WHITE MUSTARD SEED

White mustard seed has a pungent and acrid nature. It warms the lung, sweeps phlegm, and disinhibits qì; it also disperses binds, frees the network vessels, and alleviates pain. It is used to treat cold phlegm cough and panting, distention and pain of the rib-side and chest, phlegm-damp streaming sores, pain and numbness of joints, yīn flat-abscess toxin swelling, and other phlegm disorders.

RAPESEED

With a bland flavor and warm nature, rapeseed moves blood and breaks qì, disperses swelling and dissipates binds. It is used in the treatment of postpartum disorders, hemorrhoids, blood dysentery, and toxin swelling.

CUSCUTA SEED

Cuscuta seed is acrid and slightly bitter; it warms the spleen, checks diarrhea and contains spittle, and warms kidney, secures essence, and reduces urination. It is used to treat spleen-cold diarrhea with cold abdominal pain, copious spittle, kidney vacuity enuresis, frequent urination, turbid white leukorrhea, and seminal emission.

SPINY JUJUBA KERNEL

With sour and sweet taste and a warm nature, spiny jujuba kernel supplements the liver, quiets the spirit, constrains sweat, and engenders liquids. It is used to treat vacuity agitation and insomnia, fright palpitations and profuse dreaming, general vacuity and profuse sweating, and dry mouth due to damaged liquids. The seed should be cut in half, then used with the smooth surface against the ear point.

BORNEOL SEED

Borneol is an acrid-cooling medicinal; it opens the orifices and arouses the brain, clears heat, and relieves pain. It is used to treat warm diseases marked by clouded spirit, tetanic reversal, windstroke with phlegm reversal, coma, mouth sores, bloodshot eyes, and sore throat. Change treatment to the opposite ear every three days because borneol may dissolve and be absorbed in that time.

MAGNETIC BEAD ACUPRESSURE

Pressure from a 500 gauss (500G) magnetic bead can both stimulate an ear point and achieve the function of magnetic therapy. See the section later in this chapter for more details on this method.

Acupressure with Six Spirits Pill (Lìu Shén wán)

As a prepared medicine, Six Spirits Pill (*Lìu Shén Wán*) is effective for treating sore throat and tonsillitis. It is composed of bovine bezoar (*níu huáng*), musk (*shè xiāng*), toad venom (*chán sū*) pearl (*zhēn zhū*), borneol (*bīng piàn*), and realgar (*xióng huáng*); it clears heat and resolves toxins, opens the orifices and moves blood, and disperses swelling and alleviates pain. Six Spirits Pill acupressure (see p. 71) is used to treat various hot diseases and inflammation.

Needling with Filiform Needles

For this method, use half-inch, 30 gauge needles.

Procedure

Identification of Sensitive Spots

Determine the prescription according to ear diagnosis, then identify sensitive spots in selected point areas, using inspection, palpation for tenderness, and electrical detection.

Sterilization of Area to be Treated

The area to be treated or the whole auricle, if necessary, should be sterilized with 75% alcohol, particularly the triangular fossa, superior and inferior concha, and external auditory canal.

Patient Positioning

The patient generally sits down. Lying supine is acceptable for patients who feel nervous or are weak. Fix the auricle with the thumb and index finger of the non-needling hand. Place the middle finger on the posterior surface of the ear, behind the area to be needled, to control the depth of needling and relieve pain. Hold a needle with the thumb and index finger of the needling hand, and insert it into the sensitive point.

Two methods can be used for needle insertion:

Rapid Insertion: Using force, quickly insert the needle into the sensitive point in the cartilage of the ear.

Slow Insertion: Slowly insert the needle while rotating it with an even force in a clockwise direction.

INTENSITY OF STIMULATION AND MANIPULATIONS

Stimulation intensity for ear needle manipulations is determined by the individual condition of the patient, including the seriousness of the illness, age, constitution, and pain tolerance.

Intensity of Needling

The intensity of needling is clinically divided into three kinds.

Strong stimulation

This is also called draining method. It is usually used for treating acute cases, heat patterns, repletion patterns, and patients with strong constitutions.

Mild stimulation

This is also called supplementing method. It is mainly used for treating chronic conditions, vacuity patterns, and patients with weak constitutions.

Medium stimulation

This is also called even supplementation and drainage method. As the most commonly used method, it can be used in the treatment of almost all disorders.

Manipulations

The four most commonly used manipulations are: simple needling, scraping, rotating, and lifting and thrusting.

Simple needling

Insert needles into sensitive points and retain them. This is used for older adults, the weak, infants, and chronically ill patients.

Scraping

Insert needles into sensitive points, fix the inserted needles with the thumb and index finger, then quickly scrape up and down the needle handle with the nail of the thumb or finger; scrape for 20 to 30 seconds. This is commonly used for chronic diseases, a weak debilitated constitution, or for children.

Rotating

Insert the needle into the selected sensitive point, then rotate the needle with the thumb and index finger. The rotating should be done with medium intensity. Continue rotating for 20 to 30 seconds. This is suitable for treating commonly seen chronic disorders.

Lifting and Thrusting

Insert the needle into the selected sensitive point, and forcefully lift and thrust the needle in a pumping action for 10 to 20 seconds. This is used for treating acute disorders and painful disorders.

Needling Depth

The depth of needling depends on the thickness of the patient's auricle. In general, insert the needle until it reaches the ear cartilage and can stand by itself. Most practitioners think that the ear cartilage should be pierced in treating heat or repletion patterns with pain, so as to achieve strong stimulation; but the needle should be inserted only as far as the ear cartilage for those who are weak or whose illness is long-term. However, the needle should not pierce completely through the auricle, or an infection may result.

In some cases, discomfort will be relieved immediately as long as the needle is inserted and there is a needle sensation indicating qì has been obtained; if there is no needle sensation, the direction of the needle tip should be gently adjusted until the sensation is induced.

NEEDLE RETENTION AND DRAINING/SUPPLEMENTING

Needle Retention

Retention refers to keeping the needle inserted in the ear point for a period of time, generally for 30 to 60 minutes. Needle retention may be longer in chronic and painful disorders. Repeated manipulation while the needle is retained strengthens the therapeutic effect. When treating older adults or infants, retain the needles for a shorter time.

Draining and Supplementing

Draining or supplementing is achieved by the duration of the needle's retention and the intensity of stimulation. Draining refers to needling deeply while rotating, and retaining the inserted needles for a longer time. Supplementing refers to needling shallowly without rotating and retaining the inserted needles for a shorter time or not at all. Draining is generally used for treating heat and repletion patterns, or for treating pain; supplementing is used for vacuity cold patterns, weak patients, older adults, women, and infants.

NEEDLE WITHDRAWAL

Needles must be withdrawn after treatment. There are two methods for withdrawing needles.

Straight Needle Withdrawal

Fix the auricle with one hand and hold the needle handle with the thumb and index finger of the opposite hand, then withdraw the needle directly.

Because this method does not cause pain, it is frequently used in the clinic.

Rotating Needle Withdrawal

Fix the auricle with one hand while holding the needle with the thumb and index finger of the other; rotate the needle while withdrawing it.

Because stimulation is continued while withdrawing the needle, this method is generally used for heat and repletion patterns and painful disorders that require draining methods.

Press a sterilized cotton ball into the point where the needle was withdrawn to prevent bleeding and infection.

TREATMENT COURSE

Treatments are generally done daily or every other day. Allow seven to ten days for each treatment course with an interval of two or three days between treatment courses.

NEEDLE IMPLANTATION

Intradermal needles are implanted at points that treat a specific disorder. With its persistent and weak stimulation, this method is suitable for treating chronic and painful disorders, or for patients who for some reason cannot return to the clinic.

Procedure

IDENTIFICATION OF SENSITIVE POINTS

After determining the prescription according to ear diagnosis, identify sensitive points in selected areas according to inspection, tenderness, and electrical detection.

STERILIZATION

The area to be treated or, if necessary, the whole auricle should be sterilized with 75% alcohol, particularly the triangular fossa, the superior and inferior concha, and the external auditory canal.

NEEDLE INSERTION

Fix the auricle with one hand, drawing the area to be treated taut. Gently insert an intradermal needle with tweezers, then fix the inserted needle with an adhesive strip.

TREATMENT COURSE

One ear is treated first at three to five points. The patient should press the implanted needles three to five times each day, holding the pressure for two to three minutes each time. Change to the opposite ear every five to seven days. One treatment course should last ten days.

Points for Attention

- Carefully sterilize the auricle before treatment to avoid infection.

- This method cannot be used on those with ear infections or frostbite.

- Following treatment, the patient should press the implanted needles three to five times every day to improve the therapeutic effect.

- For those who have difficulty sleeping due to pain in the area where the needle is implanted, the direction of the needle tip and depth of insertion should be adjusted until the patient feels comfortable.

- Keep the area of implantation dry to avoid infection. The duration of implantation should be shorter in the summer to avoid infection.

- Local swelling and discomfort in the area of implantation should be dealt with in a timely manner. The needle should be withdrawn and anti-inflammatory treatment should be given if redness and swelling occur at the point where the intradermal needle is implanted.

ELECTROACUPUNCTURE

Electroacupuncture combines electrical stimulation with needling in order to strengthen the therapeutic effect. Almost all disorders that can be treated with ear needling can be treated with electroacupuncture, particularly psychological disorders, nervous system disorders, spasm of internal organs, and asthma.

Procedure

NEEDLE INSERTION

Insert filiform needles into the selected points in the same way as standard needling with filiform needles.

EQUIPMENT SET-UP

Connect the inserted needles to an electrical stimulator. Select the prescribed wave type and frequency, then switch on the machine and gradually increase the current to the patient's tolerance. Each treatment generally lasts ten to twenty minutes.

TREATMENT COURSE

Treat daily or every other day for seven to ten days. The treatment course may be repeated after an interval of two to three days.

Points for Attention

- The patient's condition determines the intensity of stimulation. In general, medium stimulation is used to the patient's tolerance. Stronger stimulation is used for those with severe and protracted pain.

- Connect both electrodes of one conducting wire in the same ear; set and pair electrodes separately when more than two or three needles are inserted.

- During treatment, be sure the inserted needles are not touching each other, to avoid a short circuit, which could decrease the therapeutic effect and even damage the electroacupuncture apparatus. If only one needle is used, a separate electrode can be either fixed on the rim of the auricle or held by the patient.

- Prior to treatment, inform the patient that feelings such as sleepiness, heaviness, soreness, distention, or pain are not uncommon.

- Start with a low current for several minutes, then gradually increase it.

- If the output is intermittent, it may indicate poor wire conduction. Stop the treatment and have the electroacupuncture apparatus checked and repaired before using it again.

- Regularly check the battery and other parts of the electroacupuncture apparatus to be sure they are functioning properly.

PLUM BLOSSOM NEEDLING

Plum blossom needling originated as a treatment in standard body acupuncture and was later adapted to ear acupuncture. It courses and frees the channels and network vessels, clears heat and eliminates toxins, dispels stasis and engenders new blood, and regulates the bowels and viscera.

INDICATIONS

Facial paralysis, neuritis of the lateral cutaneous nerve of the thigh, dermal disorders such as acne, rose acne, brandy nose, flat warts, seborreic dermatitis, chloasma, leukoderma, neurodermatitis, cutaneous pruritus, and facial cosmetic treatments.

Procedure

PREPARATION OF NEEDLES

Plum blossom ear needles are made by bunching five 0.5 inch filiform needles. Intradermal needles can also be used to make plum blossom needles for ear acupuncture. Plum blossom ear needles can be purchased ready-made.

NEEDLE INSERTION

The patient should massage both ears until the capillaries are well filled.

After sterilizing the ear, fix the auricle with one hand and hold the plum blossom needles with the other. Prick the selected points like a bird pecking. Gradually increase the strength of the pecking until the auricle feels hot and a few droplets of blood can be seen.

Clean the auricle with 75% alcohol after the treatment.

TREATMENT COURSE

Treatments should be done every other day or once every three or four days. One treatment course lasts seven to ten days; allow five days between treatment courses.

Points for Attention

- Examine the needles before treatment. Do not use needles with damaged tips.

- Points in the ear lobe can be used together with body points on the face and cheek for facial beauty treatments.

BLOODLETTING

Bloodletting can be done with either a three-edged needle or a small surgical knife on veins on the posterior surface of the ears. This procedure courses and frees the channels and network vessels, dispels stasis and engenders new blood, extinguishes wind and checks tetany, calms the patient and discharges heat, and relaxes tension and alleviates pain.

It is also used to treat painful patterns due to blood stasis, high fever and convulsion caused by exuberant, intense evil heat, or dizzy head and dizzy vision brought about by ascendant hyperactivity of liver yáng.

Procedure

SELECTION OF AREA TO BE TREATED

Bloodletting is usually done on the ear lobe, the ear apex, or at protruding veins in the auricle.

STERILIZATION

Sterilize the auricle with 75% alcohol, first on the medial side, then the lateral side, giving particular attention to the bloodletting areas.

METHOD

Massage the auricle until redness and heat are felt. Fix the auricle with one hand while holding a three-edged needle or surgical knife with the other; prick or cut the skin to draw three to five drops of blood, then stop the bleeding with pressure.

TREATMENT COURSE

In general, one treatment is done every other day. However, it should be done once a day for acute febrile diseases. Allow five to seven days for each treatment course with an interval of two or three days between courses.

Points for Attention

- Massage the auricle before treatment to strengthen the therapeutic effect.

- Carefully control the depth of the cuts to avoid harming the ear cartilage.

- In the patient who has bloodletting done at veins on the posterior surface of the ear, use the distal veins first. Apply pressure after drawing blood to avoid formation of a subcutaneous hematoma.

- This method cannot be used for hemophilia patients, pregnant women, or anyone using blood-thinning medications.

- Careful sterilization is needed to avoid infection.

- In general, if bloodletting is done in veins on the posterior surface of the ear, treatment is performed on a single ear and changed to the other ear at the following session.

MEDICINE INJECTION

The combination of needling and injecting small amounts of drugs into the ear points can achieve a good therapeutic result.

Selection of Medicines

Choose medicines that (1) are mildly stimulating, (2) do not cause necrosis of dermal tissues, and (3) are easily absorbed.

COMMONLY USED MEDICINES

Surface Anesthetic Agents: Novocain and Lidocaine.

Vitamins: Vitamin B$_1$, vitamin B$_{12}$ and vitamin E.

Sedatives: Phenobarbitol and chlorpromazine hydrochloride.

Antibiotics: Penicillin and Gentamicin.

Analgesics: Pethidine hydrochloride and anadolum .

Antispasmodics: Atropine sulfate and scopolamine hydrobromide.

Antiasthmatics: Epinephrine bitartrate and aminophylline.

CNS stimulants: Lobeline hydrochloride, nikethamide, strychnine, and securininum.

Hormones: Hydrocortisone and insulin.

Hemostatics: Adrenaline, salicylates, and vitamin K.

Biological Products: Placental tissue fluid and brain tissue fluid.

Herbal Medicinal Products: *Huáng Qí Zhù Shè Yè* (Astragalus Injection Fluid), *Dáng Guī Zhù Shè Yè* (Tangkue Injection Fluid), *Chái Hú Zhù Shè Yè* (Bupleurum Injection Fluid) and *Bǎn Lán Gēn Zhù Shè Yè* (Isatis Root Injection Fluid).

Normal saline and distilled water can also be used in injections.

Procedure

SELECTION OF AREA TO BE TREATED

Determine the prescription for both acupuncture points and medicines according to the diagnosis.

STERILIZATION

Sterilize the auricle with 75% alcohol.

INJECTION OF MEDICINES

Draw up the selected medicine into a syringe. Fix the auricle with one hand to make the area to be treated taut, then inject the drug with the other hand. Inject 0.1–0.5 ml of the medicine in each point until a blister is seen in the injected area. Local redness, swelling, heat, or pain may be induced.

Gently wipe away spills around the injected area. Avoid forceful pressing or kneading.

TREATMENT COURSE

Inject points in alternate ears every other day. Allow five to seven treatments for each course with an interval of two or three days between courses.

Points for Attention

- Only a small amount of a drug is needed.
- Careful sterilization is necessary to avoid infection.
- Give a skin test for any medicine that may cause an allergic reaction.
- Give adequate attention to the drug's pharmacological functions and contraindications. Avoid medicines having severe side effects or drugs that are stimulating.
- Start with a small dose and gradually increase, particularly for older adults, those who are weak, or those who have never been treated with this method.
- Use points in alternation to benefit drug absorption.

EAR MOXIBUSTION

Ear moxibustion achieves an effect of a warm and hot nature. This method warms the channels and dissipates cold, and courses and frees the channels and network vessels. It is recommended for treating vacuity cold pattern and impediment syndrome.

Procedure

MOXIBUSTION WITH INCENSE

Light an incense stick. Two or three points are selected for treatment. Hold the incense stick close to the skin for two to three minutes, until the patient feels a mild burning pain. Treat one ear each session, and alternate ears every other day. Allow seven to ten treatments for each course. This method is used to treat condititions such as pain in the lumbus and legs, crick in the neck, and periarthritis of the shoulder joint.

MOXIBUSTION WITH JUNCUS

Cut juncus into one-centimeter segments and soak in rapeseed oil to prepare for use. Light the soaked juncus and quickly moxibust the selected point until the sound "pah" is heard. This counts as one cone. Treat daily or every other day, using three to nine cones for each treatment. Whether to treat one or both ears at the same time is determined by whether the disease involves one side or both sides of the body. This method is used to treat mumps, conjunctivitis, and herpes zoster.

MOXIBUSTION WITH MATCH STICKS

Light a match stick, and then quickly press the burning stick into the selected point for one to two seconds. Treat one or two points on alternating ears.

MOXIBUSTION WITH MOXA POLE

Use a moxa pole on the whole auricle until it is reddened and a hot feeling is induced. This method is used to treat painful impediment, wilting pattern, and soreness and pain in the lumbus and knees.

Points for Attention

- Take care that hair is not burned during treatment.
- In order to avoid burns, continue moxibustion only until redness of the auricle, a heat sensation, or a mild burning pain is induced.
- Treat all selected ear points in turn.
- Moxibustion is not recommended for patients with nervousness or severe heart disease, or for infants, or pregnant women.

EAR MASSAGE

Ear massage is another method for treating ear points. A variety of massage techniques can be applied either to the entire ear or to specific points. The purpose of this therapy can be either general disease prevention or specific diseases remediation.

Procedure

Various rubbing, pinching, and kneading techniques are performed with the fingers or the palms at different areas in the ear. This method works both for treatment and prevention of diseases.

Whole Ear Massage

The practitioner should vigorously rub his palms together until heat is induced, then press his palms on the patient's auricles, rubbing up and down as well as back and forth on both the anterior and posterior surfaces of the ears; this should continue until heat and redness are induced in the patient's ears.

This method is used to treat disorders of the channels and network vessels and the bowels and viscera. Continuous daily treatments prevent diseases and strengthen the body.

Rubbing the Helix with the Palms

This method was praised in ancient China. According to ancient longevity methods, "Using the hands to rub the helix, rub as much as you can. . . . [This] supplements kidney qì to prevent deafness."

The actual method is to make loose fists with the hands, then rub up and down along the external helix of both ears with the thumb and index finger until redness of the helix and heat are induced.

By fortifying the brain, brightening the eyes, supplementing the kidney, sharpening hearing, and fortifying general health, this method can be used to treat and prevent yáng wilt, frequent and urgent urination, hemorrhoids, pain in the lumbus and legs, diarrhea, spondylopathy, oppression in the chest, dizziness, and headache.

Lifting and Pinching the Ear Lobe

Use both hands to lift while pinching both ear lobes, gradually increasing the strength of the manipulation. Treat two times per day, once in the morning and once at night, for three to five minutes per treatment.

This method can be used to treat headache, dizziness, high fever, and convulsion in infants, as well as for disorders of the eyes and for prevention of the common cold, vision and hearing enhancement, and for physical beauty.

EAR POINT MASSAGE

There are three commonly used ear-point massage methods.

Point-Pressing (diǎn àn)

With a spring stick or detection stick, **point-press** (diǎn àn) at the points related to the disorder. Using gradually increasing strength, continue *point-pressing* (*diǎn àn*) for one to two minutes until distention, heat, or a painful sensation is induced in the treated area.

This method is mainly used to treat pain disorders and prevent diseases.

Pinch Pressing (qiā àn)

Place the thumb at a selected point on the anterior surface of the ear with the index finger on the posterior surface and **pinch press** (*qiā àn*), gradually increasing the strength of the pressing. Select one to three points for each treatment.

This method is mainly used to treat pain disorders and to prevent the common cold.

Kneading–Pressing (róu àn)

Knead in a clockwise direction, using the tip of the index finger or a detection stick, until distention and heat are induced in the selected area.

This method is suitable for treating pain disorders and for poor digestion in infants, as well as for those with a sensitive constitution.

Points for Attention

- Increasing the duration of ear massage improves its therapeutic effect.
- Do not use ear massage on patients with inflammation or frostbite in the auricle.

MEDICATED PLASTERS

In this method, medicated bandages, or plasters, are affixed to the ear so that the stimulation from the medication upon the contacted ear points will treat the disease.

This method is used to treat laryngopharyngitis, cough, asthma, bronchitis, headache, dizziness, hypertension, pain in the upper abdomen, lumbus, and legs, and coronary heart disease.

TYPES OF PLASTERS

Medicinal plasters can be purchased ready-made.

Toxin-Resolving Plasters

These include *Dà Qīng Gāo* (Major Green-Blue Plaster), *Dú Jiǎo Gāo* (Single Horn Plaster), and *Bá Dú Gāo* (Toxin-Extracting Plaster). With the functions of clearing heat and resolving toxins, they are suitable for treating various febrile disorders and inflammatory conditions, particularly those occurring in infants.

Blood-Quickening Plasters

These include *Dōng Fāng Huó Xuě Gāo* (Oriental Blood-Invigorating Plaster) and *Zhèn Jiāng Gāo* (Zhen Jiang Plaster). With the functions of activating the channels and network vessels, and quickening the blood and transforming stasis, they are suitable for treating arthritis. Do not treat pregnant women with these bandages.

Pain-Alleviating Plasters

Pain-alleviating plasters include *Shāng Shī Zhǐ Tòng Gāo* (Dampness Damage Pain-Relieving Plaster), *Shè Xiāng Hǔ Gǔ Gāo* (Musk and Tiger Bone Plaster), and *Zhǐ Tòng Gāo* (Pain-Alleviating Plaster). With the functions of draining inflammation and alleviating pain, these are suitable for treating arthritis. Pregnant women and patients who are allergic to plasters should not be treated with these bandages.

Blood Pressure-Lowering Plaster

Jiàng Yā Gāo (Blood Pressure Lowering Plaster) is used to treat hypertension.

Procedure

First determine the prescription according to ear diagnosis, then identify sensitive spots within selected point areas according to inspection, tenderness, and electrical detection. Sterilize the area to be treated, or the whole auricle if necessary, with 75% alcohol. Cut the plasters into pieces 0.6 centimeters square, and apply them to the selected points.

TREATMENT COURSE

The ears can be treated together or in alternation. Change the bandages every three days. Treatment courses should be shorter during the summertime.

Points for Attention

- Choose plasters according to their functions and the patient's condition.
- Keep the plasters dry and clean.

MAGNET THERAPY

A magnetic bead or small pad is affixed to ear points to treat diseases by the effect of the magnetic force on the points.

This method settles pain, relieves itching, checks panting, and regulates autonomic nerve function.

Procedure

Sterilize the auricle with 75% alcohol to remove oils.

DIRECT MAGNET THERAPY

Place a magnetic bead or pad at the center of an adhesive strip. Then affix the prepared strip to the selected point. A second bead or pad should be affixed on the opposite side of the ear, with the opposite pole facing the first bead or pad.

INDIRECT MAGNET THERAPY

Wrap a magnetic bead or pad in a thin layer of absorbent cotton and place it at the center of an adhesive strip. The prepared strip is then affixed to the selected point and a second bead or pad is positioned on the opposite side of the ear, just as in direct magnet therapy. The layer of cotton prevents the uncomfortable stimulation and necrosis of local skin that may be caused by direct contact.

Treat deafness and tinnitus by placing a wrapped magnetic bead into the external auditory canal.

NEEDLE IMPLANTATION IN COMBINATION WITH MAGNET THERAPY

Implant needles into the prescribed points, then attach magnetic beads to the handles of the needles to conduct a magnetic field into the patient's body via the needle. Treat once a day.

This method is effective for treating dermal diseases and pain disorders.

MAGNETIC ELECTROACUPUNCTURE

Use 1000G magnetic beads. Weld beads to both the negative and positive poles of a conducting wire. Fix the welded magnetic beads at the selected points and then connect them to an electrical stimulator. Pulsed current is conducted into the body through the magnetic beads. Select one pair of electrical poles for each treatment, every other day, for 10 to 30 minutes each treatment.

This method is effective for relieving pain and settling the spirit.

MAGNETIC CLAY THERAPY

Grind a prepared mixture of magnetic rock powder, hyoscyamine, menthol, sulfamehoxypyrldazine, and berberine into powder, then add Chinese holly leaf oil to make a paste. Apply the paste to the selected points in the daytime, and wash it off at night.

Points for Attention

- Dizziness, nausea, listlessness, drowsiness, or burning or itching feeling in the treated areas may occur in 5-10% of patients who are treated with magnet therapy. Palpitations, excitement, or insomnia may occur in very few cases. All these symptoms usually disappear with no treatment in a few minutes or a few days. Discontinue treatment if the patient experiences persistent discomfort.

- Depending on a patient's condition, a combination of two or three magnet therapy methods can be used to enhance the therapeutic effect. Few points are used.

- Positive and negative poles should be placed on opposite sides of the auricle to make a line of magnetic force cross the intended ear point.

- Continue treatment for up to two weeks after all symptoms disappear to reinforce the therapeutic effect.

OTHER TREATMENT METHODS

Since the late 1950s there has been a good deal of research done in China regarding effective ways to treat ear points. In addition to the methods that have already been explained in this chapter, there has also been work done with laser therapy, radio-isotope therapy, the use of ear clips, scraping therapy, and a compound therapy method.

Briefly, laser and radio-isotope therapies try to apply these modern forces to the ear to restore health. Some doctors, especially pediatricians, bend a paper-clip-like device into a shape that applies constant pressure to an ear point. In scraping therapy, the selected points are physically scraped. In one version of compound therapy, the ears are first massaged, then bloodletting is performed, and finally the blood is reinjected at certain body acupuncture points. These therapies are mentioned only in passing as we believe they have limited use.

CHAPTER FIVE

TREATMENTS FOR COMMON DISORDERS

The case studies with comments in this section are from the clinical records of Dr. Yang Yun Bi, at the Medical School of Huang Shan (Yellow Mountain City) in Anhui Province, PRC.

INFECTIOUS DISORDERS

Common Cold

TREATMENT PRESCRIPTION

Primary Points: Lung (MA-IC1), Internal Nose (MA-T), Kidney (MA-SC), Ear Shén Mén (MA-TF1).

Supplementary Points: Ear Apex (MA-H6) and Helix 1-6 (MA-H 1-6) for fever; Forehead (MA-AT), Kidney (MA-SC), and Spleen (MA-IC) for headache and aching; Pharynx and Larynx (MA-T3) for sore throat; Bronchii/Trachea (MA-IC2) and Calm Panting (MA-AT) for cough; Stomach (MA-IC) and Spleen (MA-IC) for diarrhea and vomiting.

THERAPEUTIC METHODS

Ear Acupuncture: Select two or three primary points together with one or two supplementary points. The needles should be forcefully rotated to create intense stimulation. Two treatments per day are recommended for a severe case. Retain the needles for 30 to 60 minutes and manipulate every 10 to 15 minutes. Decrease treatments to once per day as the illness improves.

Ear Acupressure: Affix seeds to selected points in both ears. Press the seeds three to five times per day (morning, noon, afternoon, and evening), three to five minutes each time.

Bloodletting: To be used in those with fever. Ear Apex (MA-H6) and Helix 1-6 (MA-H 1-6) are treated.

NOTES

- Clinical practice shows that ear acupuncture not only treats the common cold, but can also prevent it. As a preventative measure for cases of repeated attack of the common cold due to a weak constitution or in a period of epidemic of influenza, apply ear acupuncture, ear acupressure, or massage at Lung (MA-IC1), Spleen (MA-IC), and Kidney (MA-SC).
- According to TCM, Lung (MA-IC1) diffuses the lung and resolves the exterior; it thereby frees the nose and thus is the primary point for the treatment of common cold and influenza. Kidney (MA-SC) is anti-inflammatory and anti-allergic, so it is effective for runny nose and excessive lacrimation when combined with Lung (MA-IC1). Bleeding at Ear Apex (MA-H6) and Helix 1-6 (MA-H 1-6) clears lung heat. Severe cases of influenza or pneumonic common cold should be treated with ear acupuncture in combination with other therapies.

CASE STUDY: COMMON COLD

Zhang, a 20-year-old female, reported that for two days she had headache, fever, nasal congestion with runny nose, and sore throat. Her body temperature was 38° C; there was redness and swelling in her throat. The diagnosis was "common cold."

Treatment Prescription: Ear Apex (MA-H6), Internal Nose (MA-T), Throat (MA-T3), Lung (MA-IC1), Adrenal Gland (MA-T), and Occiput (MA-AT).

Therapeutic Method: Bleeding at Ear Apex (MA-H6) with three-edged needle; seed acupressure for the other points. Both ears were treated simultaneously, twice a week. The patient was told to press the seeds three to five times per day during the treatment.

Treatment Results: The patient's body temperature returned to normal; all other symptoms showed improvement six hours after the first treatment. All the symptoms were gone after three treatments.

COMMENTS:

1. Bleeding at Ear Apex (MA-H6), usually by drawing three drops of blood, is remarkably effective for reducing body temperature.
2. In common cold, the identified patterns can change very quickly. Other therapies should be considered whenever a complication occurs.

Epidemic Parotitis/Mumps

TREATMENT PRESCRIPTION 1

Primary Points: Apex of Antitragus (MA-AT), Cheek (MA-L), Adrenal Gland (MA-T) and Ear Apex (MA-H6).

Supplementary Points: Endocrine (MA-IC3), Subcortex (MA-AT1), Stomach (MA-IC), Pancreas/Gallbladder (MA-SC6), and Ear Shén Mén (MA-TF1).

THERAPEUTIC METHOD

Ear Acupuncture: Use all the primary points together with one or two supplementary points, according to the patient's condition. The needles should be retained for 30 minutes and forcefully rotated every 10 minutes to achieve strong stimulation. Treat one or two times per day on both ears.

TREATMENT PRESCRIPTION 2

Primary Points: Parotid Gland (MA-AT), Ear Apex (MA-H6), and Ear Shén Mén (MA-TF1).

THERAPEUTIC METHOD

Ear Acupressure: Affix seeds to all prescribed points on both ears. Press the seeds three to five times per day, two to three minutes each time, until the swelling is decreased. This should occur in two to four days.

TREATMENT PRESCRIPTION 3

Primary Points: Ear Apex (MA-H6).

THERAPEUTIC METHOD

Bloodletting: Puncture Ear Apex (MA-H6) on both ears with a three-edged needle to draw ten drops of blood. Treat once per day for common cases, two treatments for severe cases.

CASE STUDY: EPIDEMIC MUMPS

Chen, a 5-year-old girl, had suffered from fever and painful swollen cheeks for three days. Her body temperature was 38° C; she had swelling and tenderness centered at the ear lobes and extending to both cheeks and surrounding area. The diagnosis was "epidemic mumps."

Treatment Prescription: Apex of Antitragus (MA-AT), Cheek (MA-L), Ear Apex (MA-H6), Adrenal Gland (MA-T), and Subcortex (MA-AT1).

Therapeutic Method: Bleeding at Ear Apex (MA-H6) with a three-edged needle. The other points were needled with filiform needles on both ears. The needles were retained for 30 minutes.

Treatment Results: Pain was greatly improved after the first treatment, and all the symptoms were gone after two treatments. The patient took no other medication or therapy during the treatment with ear acupuncture.

Comment: Considering that children are afraid of needling, seed acupressure can also be effective for the treatment of this disorder.

Whooping Cough

TREATMENT PRESCRIPTION

Primary Points: Bronchi (MA-IC), Lung (MA-IC1), Ear Shén Mén (MA-TF1), and Sympathetic (MA-AH7).

Supplementary Points: Large Intestine (MA-SC4), Ear Apex (MA-H6), Apex of Antitragus (MA-AT), Subcortex (MA-AT1), Adrenal Gland (MA-T), and Kidney (MA-SC).

THERAPEUTIC METHODS

Ear Acupuncture: Use all the primary points together with one or two supplementary points according to the patient's current condition; for example, select Ear Apex (MA-H6) and Apex of Antitragus (MA-AT) at the early stage; select Subcortex (MA-AT1) and Adrenal Gland (MA-T) at the spasmodic cough stage; and select Kidney (MA-SC) and Ear Shén Mén (MA-TF1) at the recovery stage. Rotate the inserted needles, then remove them immediately. One treatment per day is done at both the early stage and the recovery stage; treat two or three times per day at the paroxysmal cough stage. Begin treatment on a single ear and change to the opposite ear every other day. One treatment course is seven days; allow two to three days between treatment courses.

Bloodletting: After routine sterilization, draw two to three drops of blood using a sterilized three-edged needle at Ear Apex (MA-H6) every other day. This treatment is for those with fever at the early stage.

CASE STUDY: WHOOPING COUGH

Wang, a 7-year-old boy, suffered from cough for one month. The paroxysmal coughing was aggravated at night and was followed by chicken-crowing-like breathing with scanty white foamy sputum. Sometimes when the cough was severe it resulted in vomiting. The boy also had congestion of the bulbar conjunctiva in both eyes and a slightly puffy face. Auscultation revealed rough breathing on both sides of the lung. An X-ray exam showed no other diseases in the lungs. The diagnosis was "whooping cough."

Treatment Prescription: Bronchii/Trachea (MA-IC2), Lung (MA-IC1), Adrenal Gland (MA-T), Mouth (MA-IC5), and Central Rim (MA-AT).

> **Therapeutic Method:** The initial treatment selection was needling at the above points on both ears.
>
> **Treatment Results:** The patient's cough was remarkably improved the very night of the first treatment. Seed acupressure was used from the second treatment on the following day; both ears were treated once per day. All the symptoms were gone after seven treatments, and one more treatment was added to strengthen the therapeutic effect.
>
> **Comment:** Ear acupuncture is better for whooping cough at late stage marked by dry cough because it can reduce the sensitivity of new epifollicles in the trachea and bronchus, as well as inhibit the respiratory center in the brain stem.

Tuberculosis

TREATMENT PRESCRIPTION 1

Primary Points: Lung (MA-IC1), Endocrine (MA-IC3), and Ear Shén Mén (MA-TF1).

Supplementary Points: Chest (MA-AH11), Kidney (MA-SC), Spleen (MA-IC), Stomach (MA-IC), Internal Reproductive Organs (MA-TF), and Pelvis (MA-TF).

THERAPEUTIC METHODS

Ear Acupuncture: Use all the primary points together with one or two supplementary points depending on the patient's condition. For example, add Chest (MA-AH11) and Kidney (MA-SC) for cough and chest pain; add Spleen (MA-IC) and Stomach (MA-IC) for poor appetite; add Internal Reproductive Organs (MA-TF) and Pelvis (MA-TF) for irregular menstrual cycle and amenorrhea. Manipulate by needle scratching or rotation the inserted needles, using mild stimulation. Treat once per day. Begin treatment on a single ear and change to the opposite ear every other day. One treatment course is ten days; allow two or three days between treatment courses.

Ear Acupressure: Affix whole round mung beans at all prescribed points. Press three to five times each day, two to three minutes each time. Begin treatment on a single ear and change to the opposite ear every five to seven days.

TREATMENT PRESCRIPTION 2

Primary Points: Lung (MA-IC1), Endocrine (MA-IC3), Ear Shén Mén (MA-TF1), Heart (MA-IC), Spleen (MA-IC), Subcortex (MA-AT1), and Kidney (MA-SC).

THERAPEUTIC METHOD

Medicine Injection: Inject 0.1 ml of 0.75% Novocain or 5–10 mg isoniazid into one or two points to make soybean-sized bumps. Begin treatment on a single ear and change to the opposite ear every other day. Treat once per day; a single treatment course is three months.

NOTES

- Verify that the needle is not inserted into a blood vessel by drawing back the syringe to check for blood before injecting the medicine into the points.
- This disease requires long-term treatment.

Hepatitis

TREATMENT PRESCRIPTION 1

Primary Points: Liver (MA-SC5), Pancreas/Gallbladder (MA-SC6), Spleen (MA-IC), and Stomach (MA-IC).

Supplementary Points: Add Pancreas/Gallbladder (MA-SC6) and Abdomen (MA-AH) for poor appetite; add Ear Shén Mén (MA-TF1) and Subcortex (MA-AT1) for pain in the right upper abdomen; add Large Intestine (MA-SC4) and Pancreas/Gallbladder (MA-SC6) for distention of the abdomen; add Heart (MA-IC), Ear Shén Mén (MA-TF1), and Subcortex (MA-AT1) for insomnia; add Liver Yáng (MA-H) and Ear Apex (MA-H6) to reduce the amount of SGPT and SGOP[9].

THERAPEUTIC METHODS

Ear Acupuncture: Select four to six points and apply needle rotation and scratching. Retain the needles for 60 minutes and manipulate them every ten to fifteen minutes. Treat once per day. Begin treatment on a single ear and change to the opposite ear every other day. One treatment course is seven to ten days; allow two or three days between treatment courses.

Medicine Injection: Use two or three points for each treatment. Inject 0.1 ml of 0.5% Novocain and 0.2–0.5 ml of vitamin B_{12} into the prescribed points. Begin treatment on a single ear and change to the opposite ear every other day. One treatment course is ten days.

TREATMENT PRESCRIPTION 2

Primary Points: Liver (MA-SC5), Pancreas/Gallbladder (MA-SC6), Spleen (MA-IC), Stomach (MA-IC), *Sān Jiāo* (MA-IC4), and Ear Center (MA-H1).

---

[9] These are measures of particular liver functions.

Supplementary Points: Use Ear Apex (MA-H6) for bloodletting; add Liver Yáng (MA-H) and Abdomen (MA-AH) for distention of the abdomen; add Bladder (MA-SC8), Ear Shén Mén (MA-TF1), and Chest (MA-AH11) for pain near the liver.

THERAPEUTIC METHODS

Electroacupuncture: Select two or three primary points together with one or two supplementary points. After sterilizing the auricle, insert filiform needles into the selected points. Then connect the needles to an electroacupuncture apparatus for 30 minutes at a setting that causes the patient to feel soreness, numbness, and distention. Treat once per day. Begin treatment on a single ear and change to the opposite ear every other day. One treatment course is ten days.

Ear Acupressure: Select two or three primary points together with one or two supplementary points. Affix vaccaria seeds at the selected points. Press the seeds after each meal and before going to sleep; rub for two to three minutes each time or until soreness, numbness, or distention is induced.

Bacillary Dysentery/Dysentery

TREATMENT PRESCRIPTION

Primary Points: Large Intestine (MA-SC4), Rectum (MA-H2), and Sympathetic (MA-AH7).

Supplementary Points: Add Ear Apex (MA-H6) and Adrenal Gland (MA-T) for high fever; add Spleen (MA-IC) and Stomach (MA-IC) for severe abdominal pain and diarrhea.

THERAPEUTIC METHODS

Ear Acupuncture: Select two or three primary points together with one or two supplementary points. Treat both ears, using strong stimulation by forcefully rotating. Retain the needles for 60 minutes and manipulate every 10 or 15 minutes. Treat once per day for mild cases, twice per day for severe cases.

Medicine Injection: Inject 0.1 ml of syntomycin, vitamin B_1, or Novocain at two or three of the prescribed points, once per day. Begin treatment on a single ear and change to the opposite ear every other day until diarrhea stops. One more injection should be given after bacterial culture results are normal. Atropine sulfate can also be used for the medicine injection method. Treat Ear Shén Mén (MA-TF1), Sympathetic (MA-AH7), and Large Intestine (MA-SC4) bilaterally; add Rectum (MA-H2) for tenesmus. Inject 0.15 ml for each point, and treat once or twice per day.

Needle Implantation: Select three to five of the points in one ear for needle implantation. Press the implanted needles two or three times per day, two to three minutes each time. The intradermal needles should remain implanted for five to seven days. In general, all signs of illness will disappear after only one treatment course.

NOTES

* Patients with toxic types of bacillary dysentery with severe manifestations should be treated on an inpatient basis using a combination of therapies.

Malaria

TREATMENT PRESCRIPTION

Primary Points: Adrenal Gland (MA-T), Subcortex (MA-AT1), and Endocrine (MA-IC3).

THERAPEUTIC METHODS

Ear Acupuncture: Select all prescribed points in both ears, using strong stimulation by rotating forcefully. Needling should be done seven hours before an attack, and the needles should be retained until one to two hours after the attack ends; manipulate the needles every 15 to 20 minutes.

Needle Implantation: Implant needles at the prescribed points in both ears two hours before an attack occurs. Press the implanted needles three to five times each day, three to five minutes each time. The needles should remain implanted until two or three days after the attacks stop.

NOTES

* Cerebral malaria and severe cases of malaria must be treated with a combination of therapies at an inpatient clinic.

INTERNAL DISORDERS

Bronchitis

TREATMENT PRESCRIPTION 1

Primary Points: Lung (MA-IC1), Bronchii/Trachea (MA-IC2), and Ear Shén Mén (MA-TF1).

Supplementary Points: Add Adrenal Gland (MA-T) and Root of Ear Vagus (MA-PS) for acute bronchitis; add Spleen (MA-IC) and Kidney (MA-SC) for chronic bronchitis; add Calm Panting (MA-AT) for pulmonary emphysema.

THERAPEUTIC METHODS

Ear Acupuncture: Select two or three primary points together with one or two supplementary points. Retain the needles for 30 to 60 minutes and manipulate every 10 to 15 minutes, use needle rotation for strong stimulation. Treat once per day. Begin treatment on a single ear and change to the opposite ear every other day. One treatment course is five to seven days; allow two or three days between treatment courses.

Ear Acupressure: Affix seeds at three to five prescribed points. Press the seeds three to five times per day, two to three minutes each time. Begin treatment on a single ear and change to the opposite ear after five to seven days. This method is mainly used to treat chronic bronchitis.

TREATMENT PRESCRIPTION 2

Primary Points: Lung (MA-IC1), Kidney (MA-SC), Calm Panting (MA-AT), and Bronchii/Trachea (MA-IC2).

THERAPEUTIC METHOD

Medicine Injection: Select one or two of the prescribed points, and inject a prepared bacteria concoction.[10] Use 0.05–0.1 ml for the first injection, gradually increasing the amount to 0.3 ml. Treat two times per week. One treatment course is ten treatments.

CASE STUDY: BRONCHITIS

Yao, a 20-year-old male, reported that for five days he had cough with frothy sputum, which was aggravated at night. After treatment with Western medication, the amount of sputum was remarkably reduced but the cough had not significantly improved. The patient's body temperature was normal. Auscultation revealed rough breath on both sides of the lung, and an X-ray exam showed no other diseases in the lungs. The diagnosis was "acute bronchitis."

Treatment Prescription: Bronchii/Trachea (MA-IC2), Lung (MA-IC1), Ear Shén Mén (MA-TF1), Mouth (MA-IC5), Central Rim (MA-AT), and Endocrine (MA-IC3).

Therapeutic Method: In the first treatment, both ears were needled and the needles were retained for 30 minutes. Seed acupressure was used starting with the second treatment.

Treatment Results: The cough was remarkably improved at night after the first treatment, and the patient was cured after three treatments.

Comments: 1. Ear acupuncture is more effective for bronchitis in an early stage or when dry cough with inflammation is under control.

---

[10] This concoction is a type of complex bacterial vaccine that combines hay bacillus with streptococcus and staphylococcus albus.

> 2. Chronic bronchitis is frequently complicated with inflammation, and ear acupuncture can only provide symptomatic relief and shorten the course of illness. For better therapeutic results, other complementary therapies should be used.

Bronchial Asthma/Wheezing and Panting

TREATMENT PRESCRIPTION

Primary Points: Lung (MA-IC1), Kidney (MA-SC), Ear Shén Mén (MA-TF1), Adrenal Gland (MA-T), and Sympathetic (MA-AH7).

Supplementary Points: Add Bronchii/Trachea (MA-IC2) for severe cough; add Chest (MA-AH11) and Subcortex (MA-AT1) for severe panting.

THERAPEUTIC METHODS

Medicine Injection: Use 0.2% Novocain or 1:1000 adrenaline. Select two or three prescribed points and inject 0.1 ml of the preparation into each point. This method is recommended for acute cases.

Ear Acupuncture: Use all primary points, together with one or two supplementary points. Retain the needles for 30 to 60 minutes and manipulate every 10 to 15 minutes, using needle scratching and rotation manipulation. Treat once per day. Begin treatment on a single ear and change to the opposite each every other day. One treatment course is seven days.

Ear Acupressure: Use white mustard seed. Rub seeds three to five times per day, two to three minutes each time. Begin treatment on a single ear and change to the opposite ear every five to seven days.

NOTE

• Ear acupressure is used as a preventative treatment during intervals between acute attacks of asthma.

CASE STUDY: BRONCHIAL ASTHMA

For the last 8 years Wang, a 19-year-old male, had suffered from asthma that was triggered by seasonal changes, catching cold, and overwork. Two days prior to his first treatment, he had sudden onset of asthma marked by difficult breathing, white frothy sputum, slightly purple lips, and wheezing sounds on both sides of the chest. The diagnosis was "bronchial asthma."

Treatment Prescription: Bronchii/Trachea (MA-IC2), Lung (MA-IC1), Kidney (MA-SC), Sympathetic (MA-AH7), Adrenal Gland (MA-T), Subcortex (MA-AT1), and Endocrine (MA-IC3).

Therapeutic Method: All the above points were needled on both ears; later, seed acupressure was used.

> **Treatment Results:** The asthma was significantly relieved within two hours of the first treatment. At the second treatment on the following day and thereafter, seed acupressure was used; treatments switched between ears every three to five days. All the symptoms were gone after four treatments.
>
> **Comments:** 1. Ear acupuncture can only relieve the symptoms at the acute onset of asthma by relaxing spasms of the bronchial smooth muscle. It does not help for complete healing.
>
> 2. As for bronchial asthma complicated with infection, an anti-inflammatory medicinal treatment should be added.

Hypertension

TREATMENT PRESCRIPTION 1

Primary Points: Groove of Posterior Surface (MA-PS), Liver (MA-SC5), and Spleen (MA-IC).

THERAPEUTIC METHOD

Bloodletting: Draw five to ten drops of blood from each of the prescribed points. Begin treatment on a single ear and change to the opposite ear every other session. For the best effect, treatment should continue every two or three days, even after blood pressure returns to normal.

NOTES

• Blood pressure may rise at the beginning of treatment in some patients, but it will gradually decline.

TREATMENT PRESCRIPTION 2

Primary Points: Adrenal Gland (MA-T), Sympathetic (MA-AH7), Heart (MA-IC), and Ear Shén Mén (MA-TF1).

Supplementary Points: Liver (MA-SC5), Kidney (MA-SC), Endocrine (MA-IC3), and Subcortex (MA-AT1).

THERAPEUTIC METHODS

Magnet Therapy: Use all the primary points together with one or two supplementary points. Select magnetic beads with a diameter of 1.5 to 2.0 mm and a magnetic intensity of 0.05 to 0.08 teslae (500 to 800G). Affix the beads onto the selected points. Begin treatment on a single ear and change to the opposite ear every five to seven days.

Ear Acupressure: Affix vaccaria seeds on two or three primary points together with one or two supplementary points. Press three to five times per day, two to three minutes each time. Begin treatment on a single ear and change to the opposite ear every five to seven days.

CASE STUDY: HYPERTENSION

Li, a 56-year-old female, had suffered from dizziness, insomnia, and hypertension (Phase I) for the last 8 years. Her blood pressure was normally in the range of 180-170/115-100 mm/Hg when she was taking hypertension medication.

Treatment Prescription: Ear Apex (MA-H6), Heart (MA-IC), Ear Shén Mén (MA-TF1), Sympathetic (MA-AH7), Hypertension (MA-TF), Groove of Posterior Surface (MA-PS), and Anterior Ear Lobe (MA-L).

Therapeutic Method: Bleed three to five drops of blood at Ear Apex (MA-H6); seed acupressure for all other points. Switch ears every three days. The patient was told to press the seeds three to five times per day during the treatment.

Treatment Results: The patient's blood pressure came down to 140/80 mm/Hg after the third treatment, and her sleep returned to normal. After seed acupressure was applied for another three months, the symptoms were all relieved and her blood pressure had stabilized in the normal range.

Comments: 1. Treatment of hypertension with ear acupuncture can achieve good therapeutic results for patients in Phase I and Phase II, but not for Phase III.

2. Other therapies should be added if three consecutive acupuncture treatments provide no relief.

3. In hypertension patients with severe headache, bleeding three drops of blood from Helix Point (located at the point 2/3 of the distance from the upper helix to the lower helix) relieves pain and brightens the eyes. But this technique does not reduce blood pressure.

Hypotension

TREATMENT PRESCRIPTION 1

Primary Points: *Shēng Yā Gōu* Blood Pressure-Raising Groove (MA-PS), a groove behind the ear lobe below the posterior groove of the superior anithelix crus.[11]

THERAPEUTIC METHOD

Ear Acupuncture: Quickly insert the needle pointing upward into the prescribed point. Twirl in only one direction until it is firmly in place and the patient feels an overall heat, distention, and pain in the auricle.

---

[11] The same point is also called *Jiàng Yā Gōu* when the blood pressure needs to be lowered. Different effects are achieved by the direction of needle insertion. Upward needling raises blood pressure, downward needling lowers blood pressure.

Retain the needle for 30 minutes and manipulate every 10 minutes. Treat once per day; seven to ten days per treatment course.

TREATMENT PRESCRIPTION 2

Primary Points: Ear Shén Mén (MA-TF1), Sympathetic (MA-AH7), Heart (MA-IC), Endocrine (MA-IC3), and Subcortex (MA-AT1).

THERAPEUTIC METHOD

Ear Acupressure: Select all the primary points. Affix vaccaria seeds and press them three to five times per day, two to three minutes each time. Begin treatment on a single ear and change to the opposite ear every five to seven days.

NOTES

- Ear acupuncture treats hypotension by improving the symptoms and raising blood pressure.
- Nodes or pitting can be found at some points such as Heart (MA-IC) and Ear Shén Mén (MA-TF1) in patients with hypotension.

CASE STUDY: HYPOTENSION

Qian, a 53-year-old female, had suffered from dizziness, lassitude, listlessness, poor appetite, insomnia, and hypotension for the last eight years. Her blood pressure was 80/50 mm/Hg. A physical examination revealed no explanation for this problem. The diagnosis was "hypotension."

Treatment Prescription: Heart (MA-IC), Kidney (MA-SC), Sympathetic (MA-AH7), Adrenal Gland (MA-T), Central Rim (MA-AT), and Subcortex (MA-AT1).

Therapeutic Method: Seed acupressure on all the above points, switching ears every three days. The patient was told to press the seeds three to five times per day during the treatment.

Treatment Results: The patient's blood pressure increased to 105-90/70-60 mm/Hg after the third treatment, and her sleep and appetite returned to normal. She continued this treatment for six months; the symptoms were all relieved and her blood pressure had stabilized in the normal range.

Comment: The above therapy is effective for stabilizing blood pressure in menopausal patients.

Sequelae of Cerebrovascular Accident

TREATMENT PRESCRIPTION

Primary Points: Subcortex (MA-AT1), Liver (MA-SC5), Kidney (MA-SC), and Spleen (MA-IC).

Supplementary Points: In general, select points according to the location of the affected areas. For example, add *Sān Jiāo* (MA-IC4), Large Intestine (MA-SC4), and Lung (MA-IC1) for muscles in an affected shoulder; add Clavicle (MA-SF5), Shoulder (MA-SF4), and Elbow (MA-SF3) for muscles in an affected upper extremity; add Hip (MA-AH4), Knee (MA-AH3), and Ankle (MA-AH2) for muscles in an affected lower extremity; add Heart (MA-IC) and Spleen (MA-IC) for aphasia; add Mouth (MA-IC5), Parynx and Larynx (MA-T3), and Root of Ear Vagus (MA-PS) for difficulty swallowing.

THERAPEUTIC METHODS

Ear Acupressure: Select two or three primary points together with one or two supplementary points. Use white mustard seeds, pressing the seeds three to five times each day, two to three minutes each time. Begin treatment on a single ear and change to the opposite ear every five to seven days.

Ear Acupuncture or Electroacupuncture: Select three to five prescribed points; insert needles to the depth of the ear perichondrium and rotate or scratch the needles. Retain the needles for 30 to 60 minutes and manipulate every 10 to 15 minutes. Treat once per day. Begin treatment on a single ear and change to the opposite ear every other day. One treatment course is ten days.

The selected points can also be connected to an electroacupuncture apparatus for 30 minutes, once a day. Ten days is a single treatment course; allow two or three days between treatment courses.

NOTES

- The earlier this disorder is treated with ear acupuncture, the more effective the treatment.
- Nodules, red spots, or pitting can be found at Subcortex (MA-AT1), Liver (MA-SC5), Kidney (MA-SC), and other points.

Post-Wind Stroke Edema

TREATMENT PRESCRIPTION

Primary Points: Spleen (MA-IC), Liver (MA-SC5), *Sān Jiāo* (MA-IC4), Wrist (MA-SF2), and Finger (MA-SF1).

THERAPEUTIC METHOD

Ear Acupressure: Select three to five of the prescribed points. Affix vaccaria seeds and press them three to five times per day, three to five minutes each time. Begin treatment on a single ear and change to the opposite ear every five to seven days.

Transient Ischemic Attack

TREATMENT PRESCRIPTION

Primary Points: Liver (MA-SC5), Kidney (MA-SC), Spleen (MA-IC), Occiput (MA-AT), and Temple (MA-AT).

Supplementary Points: Add Heart (MA-IC) and Tongue (MA-L) for difficulty in speaking; add Shoulder (MA-SF4), Elbow (MA-SF3), Knee (MA-AH3), and Hip (MA-AH4) on the contralateral side [i.e., for motor problems on the right side of the body, treat the left ear]; for limited range of motion; add Forehead (MA-AT), Ear Shén Mén (MA-TF1), and Subcortex (MA-AT1) for sensory disturbance.

THERAPEUTIC METHODS

Needle Implantation: Select two or three primary points together with one or two supplementary points; quickly implant needles into the selected points and fix the needles with an adhesive strip. Press three to five times per day, two to three minutes each time. Additionally, continue pressing the implanted needles during an attack until all signs are relieved. Begin treatment on a single ear and change to the opposite ear every five to seven days.

Ear Acupressure: Select three to five primary points together with one or two supplementary points. Affix vaccaria seeds and press them three to five times per day, two to three minutes each time. Increase both the frequency and duration of ear acupressure for severe cases. Begin treatment on a single ear and change to the opposite ear every five to seven days.

Coronary Heart Disease

TREATMENT PRESCRIPTION 1

Primary Points: Group 1 includes Sympathetic (MA-AH7), Ear Shén Mén (MA-TF1), Heart (MA-IC), Subcortex (MA-AT1), and Kidney (MA-SC). Group 2 includes Lung (MA-IC1), Spleen (MA-IC), Endocrine (MA-IC3), and Adrenal Gland (MA-T). Use one group of points for a full treatment course and alternate groups each treatment course.

THERAPEUTIC METHODS

Ear Acupressure: Use vaccaria seeds at the prescribed points in Group 1. Press the seeds three to five times per day, three to five minutes each time. Change to the points in Group 2 every five to seven days, then change to the other ear and repeat starting with Group 1 points.

Ear Acupuncture: Needle the points in Group 1 first. Retain the needles for 30 to 60 minutes and manipulate every 10 to 15 minutes. Treat once per day. Change to the points in Group 2 every five to seven days, then change to the other ear and repeat starting with Group 1 points.

TREATMENT PRESCRIPTION 2

Primary Points: Heart (MA-IC), Chest (MA-AH11), Ear Shén Mén (MA-TF1), Subcortex (MA-AT1), and Adrenal Gland (MA-T).

THERAPEUTIC METHOD

Laser Irradiation: Select two or three prescribed points, and irradiate for two to three minutes at each point. Treat once per day; one treatment course is seven days.

NOTES

- Ear acupuncture is especially effective in treating and preventing coronary heart disease and significantly improves electrocardiogram results.
- Red or gray spots can be found at Heart (MA-IC), Chest (MA-AH11), and Sympathetic (MA-AH7) in patients with this disease.

CASE STUDY: CORONARY HEART DISEASE

Xiao, a 50-year-old female, had suffered for the last 5 years from frequent attacks of angina pectoris with oppression in the chest, shortness of breath, pale face, and thready, weak, and uneven pulse. She had not been able to work for a few years. The diagnosis was "coronary heart disease."

Treatment Prescription: Heart (MA-IC), Small Intestine (MA-SC2), Kidney (MA-SC), Sympathetic (MA-AH7), Central Rim (MA-AT), and Subcortex (MA-AT1).

Therapeutic Method: Seed acupressure for all the above points. Switch ears every three days. The patient was told to press the seeds three to five times per day during the treatment.

Treatment Results: The frequency and severity of angina pectoris attacks were reduced after four treatments. After 10 treatments the patient returned to part-time work with all symptoms relieved.

Comments: 1. Because this therapy can significantly improve heart function, it can be used to treat all types of heart diseases. It usually relieves symptoms but without a remarkable improvement showing in ECG results.

2. To treat heart diseases with irregular heart beat, add *Nèi Guān* (Inner Pass, PC-6) for a better therapeutic result.

Myocardial Ischemia

TREATMENT PRESCRIPTION

Primary Points: Heart (MA-IC), Lung (MA-IC1), Liver (MA-SC5), Kidney (MA-SC), and Ear Shén Mén (MA-TF1).

THERAPEUTIC METHOD

Ear Acupressure: Select three to five prescribed points. Affix vaccaria seeds and press them three to five times per day, three to five minutes each time. Begin treatment on a single ear and change to the opposite ear every five to seven days.

Arrhythmia

TREATMENT PRESCRIPTION

Primary Points: Heart (MA-IC), Sympathetic (MA-AH7), and Ear Shén Mén (MA-TF1).

Supplementary Points: Add Small Intestine (MA-SC2) and Root of Ear Vagus (MA-PS) for organic pathological changes; add Kidney (MA-SC) and Subcortex (MA-AT1) for insomnia; add Endocrine (MA-IC3) and Subcortex (MA-AT1) for endocrine system dysfunction; add Groove of Posterior Surface (MA-PS) for hypertension.

THERAPEUTIC METHODS

Needle Implantation: Select all primary points together with one or two of the most sensitive supplementary points. Press the implanted needles three to five times per day, two to three minutes each time. Begin treatment on a single ear and change to the opposite ear every five to seven days.

Ear Acupressure: Use vaccaria seeds at all prescribed points. Press the seeds three to five times per day, three to five minutes each time. Begin treatment on a single ear and change to the opposite ear every five to seven days.

Laser Irradiation: Select three to five prescribed points and irradiate for three to five minutes each day. Treat both ears simultaneously. One treatment course is seven to ten days; allow two or three days between treatment courses.

NOTES

- All kinds of arrhythmia can be treated with ear acupuncture (regardless of whether the heartbeat is rapid or slow) because it has the capacity of bidirectional adjustment.

Rheumatic Heart Disease

TREATMENT PRESCRIPTION

Primary Points: There are two groups of points. Group 1 includes Small Intestine (MA-SC2), Subcortex (MA-AT1), Heart (MA-IC), and Ear

Shén Mén (MA-TF1). Group 2 includes Heart (MA-IC), Adrenal Gland (MA-T), Chest (MA-AH11), and Rheumatic Line (MA-SF).[12]

THERAPEUTIC METHODS

Ear Acupuncture: Use the points in Group 1. Treat both ears simultaneously in those with a good constitution. Every seven to ten days, change to the opposite group of points. For those with a weak constitution, begin treatment on a single ear, and change to the opposite ear every treatment course (seven to ten days). Treat once per day and retain the needles for 30 to 60 minutes; manipulate every 10 to 15 minutes.

Ear Acupressure: Affix vaccaria seeds on all the points in Group 1. Begin treatment in the left ear and change to Group 2 points after five to seven days (one treatment course). Change to the right ear following the second treatment course, and repeat the procedure. Press the seeds three to five times each day, three to five minutes each time.

NOTES

- Rheumatic Line (MA-SF) is the whole line between the scaphoid fossa and the antihelix.
- Ear acupuncture has proved to be particularly effective in treating rheumatic heart disease, but the duration of treatment is usually more than three months.

Viral Myocarditis

TREATMENT PRESCRIPTION

Primary Points: Heart (MA-IC), Ear Shén Mén (MA-TF1), Adrenal Gland (MA-T), Small Intestine (MA-SC2), Endocrine (MA-IC3), and Chest (MA-AH11).

THERAPEUTIC METHODS

Ear Acupuncture: In acute or subacute cases, use all the prescribed points and treat both ears simultaneously. Apply strong stimulation by needle rotation. Retain the needles for 30 to 60 minutes and manipulate every 10 to 15 minutes. Treat once or twice each day. In chronic cases, begin treatment on a single ear and change to the opposite ear every seven days (one treatment course). Treat once per day. Use needle rotation and

---

[12] Rheumatic Line is also useful for arthritic conditions of the joints. Rheumatism of the finger, wrist, elbow, shoulder, clavicle, toe, heel, ankle, knee, hip, vertebrae, chest, neck—the anatomical areas having correspondences on the antihelix and scaphoid fossa—can be alleviated by selecting that portion of the Rheumatic Line nearest to the area corresponding to the afflicted anatomy.

scratching; retain the needles for 30 minutes and manipulate every 10 minutes.

Ear Acupressure: Use three to five prescribed points. Press the vaccaria seeds three to five times each day, two to three minutes each time. Begin treatment on a single ear and change to the opposite ear every five to seven days.

Laser Irradiation: Select two or three of the prescribed points in both ears and irradiate for three to five minutes each day. One treatment course is seven days; allow two or three days between treatment courses.

Hyperlipidemia

TREATMENT PRESCRIPTION

Primary Points: Stomach (MA-IC), *Sān Jiāo* (MA-IC4), Small Intestine (MA-SC2), and Heart (MA-IC).

Supplementary Points: Pancreas/Gallbladder (MA-SC6) and Liver (MA-SC5).

THERAPEUTIC METHOD

Ear Acupressure: Select two or three primary points together with one or two supplementary points. Press the seeds three to five times per day, two to three minutes each time. Begin treatment on a single ear and change to the opposite ear every five to seven days.

NOTES

• Those diagnosed with hyperlipidemia should increase exercise time, control intake of sugar, avoid a high calorie diet, and reduce weight.

• Red spots or a red line can be seen at Stomach (MA-IC), *Sān Jiāo* (MA-IC4), and Pancreas/Gallbladder (MA-SC6) in patients with hyperlipidemia.

Gastritis

TREATMENT PRESCRIPTION 1

Primary Points: Stomach (MA-IC), Ear Shén Mén (MA-TF1), and Ear Apex (MA-H6).

Supplementary Points: Spleen (MA-IC), Large Intestine (MA-SC4).

THERAPEUTIC METHOD

Ear Acupuncture: Use all the primary points together with supplementary points, according to the patient's condition. Insert the needles using strong stimulation by lifting and thrusting and needle rotation until the predominant signs significantly subside. Retain the needles 30 to 60 minutes and manipulate every 10 to 15 minutes. Treat two times each day.

TREATMENT PRESCRIPTION 2

Primary Points: Stomach (MA-IC), Spleen (MA-IC), Lung (MA-IC1), and Sympathetic (MA-AH7).

Supplementary Points: Ear Apex (MA-H6), Kidney (MA-SC), *Sān Jiāo* (MA-IC4), Pancreas/Gallbladder (MA-SC6), Liver (MA-SC5), Ear Shén Mén (MA-TF1), and Subcortex (MA-AT1).

THERAPEUTIC METHODS

Medicine Injection: Use Vitamin B_{12} adding thiamine Chinese angelica root injection, red sage root injection, as needed. Inject into two or three prescribed points. Treat both ears simultaneously, once per week.

Ear Acupressure: Affix vaccaria seeds at all primary points together with one or two supplementary points. Press them three to five times per day, two to three minutes each time. Begin treatment on a single ear and change to the opposite ear every five to seven days.

CASE STUDY: GASTRIC NEUROSIS

Yang, a 30-year-old female, had suffered from poor appetite and from vomiting after eating for the last ten days. She had recently experienced exhaustion due to the death of her parents and from overwork. A physical examination revealed no explanation for the problem. The diagnosis was "gastric neurosis."

Treatment Prescription: Stomach (MA-IC), Spleen (MA-IC), Liver (MA-SC5), Heart (MA-IC), Subcortex (MA-AT1), and Ear Shén Mén (MA-TF1).

Therapeutic Method: Seed acupressure was used, twice a week. Both ears were alternately treated. The patient was told to press the seeds before each meal and whenever she was nauseous.

Treatment Results: Vomiting was remarkably relieved after the first two treatments, and the patient's appetite was improving. All the symptoms were gone after a total of four treatments.

Comment: Building patient confidence in ear acupuncture is helpful for increasing therapeutic effect.

Gastroduodenal Ulcer

TREATMENT PRESCRIPTION 1

Primary Points: Stomach (MA-IC), Duodenum (MA-SC1), Sympathetic (MA-AH7), and Ear Shén Mén (MA-TF1).

Supplementary Points: Add Mouth (MA-IC5), Liver (MA-SC5), Kidney (MA-SC), and Root of Ear Vagus (MA-PS) for spleen-stomach vacuity cold type; add *Sān Jiāo* (MA-IC4) and Subcortex (MA-AT1) for liver-stomach disharmony type; add Groove of Posterior Surface (MA-PS) for hemorrhage in stomach.

THERAPEUTIC METHODS

Ear Acupuncture: Use all the primary points together with one to three supplementary points. Insert the needles to the depth of the perichondrium of the ear with strong stimulation using lifting and thrusting and needle rotation. Retain the needles 30 to 60 minutes and manipulate every 10 to 15 minutes. Begin treatment on a single ear and change to the opposite ear every other day. One treatment is given per day, with five to seven days for each treatment course. Allow two or three days between treatment courses.

Ear Acupressure: Use vaccaria seeds at three to five primary points together with supplementary points as needed. Press the seeds three to five times each day, two to three minutes each time. Begin treatment on a single ear and change to the opposite ear every five to seven days.

TREATMENT PRESCRIPTION 2

Primary Points: Stomach (MA-IC) and both veins of the posterior surface of the ear.

THERAPEUTIC METHOD

Bloodletting: Draw three to five drops of blood per point with a three-edged needle every other day until hemorrhaging in the stomach stops.

Medicine Injection: Inject vitamin K_3 and carbazochrome salicylate, 0.1–0.2 ml for each point. Treat once per day. Begin treatment on a single ear and change to the opposite ear every other day.

TREATMENT PRESCRIPTION 3

Primary Points: Stomach (MA-IC), Mouth (MA-IC5), Root of Ear Vagus (MA-PS), and Liver (MA-SC5).

THERAPEUTIC METHOD

Moxibustion: Treat once per day using an incense stick for five to ten minutes at each point. Begin treatment on a single ear and change to the opposite ear every five to seven days.

NOTES

- Prescription 1 is for treating gastroduodenal ulcers marked by severe pain in the upper abdomen.
- Prescription 2 treats hemorrhage of the stomach.
- Prescription 3 treats spleen-stomach vacuity cold pattern.

Gastroptosis

TREATMENT PRESCRIPTION

Primary Points: Spleen (MA-IC), Stomach (MA-IC), Ear Shén Mén (MA-TF1), and Subcortex (MA-AT1).

THERAPEUTIC METHODS

Ear Acupressure: Affix radish seeds to three or four primary points. Press the seeds three to five times each day, two to three minutes each time. Change to the opposite ear every five to seven days.

Ear Acupuncture: Use all the primary points. Insert needles to the perichondrium using needle scratching and rotation. Retain the needles 30 minutes and manipulate every 10 minutes. Treat once per day. Begin treatment on a single ear and change to the opposite ear every other day. One treatment course is seven days; allow two or three days between treatment courses.

NOTES

- Exercises will improve the tensile force of abdominal muscles; proper food intake is essential in healing this disease.
- White spots or trophic skin at Spleen (MA-IC) and Stomach (MA-IC) may be found in those with gastroptosis.

Chronic Nonspecific Ulcerative Colitis

TREATMENT PRESCRIPTION

Primary Points: Large Intestine (MA-SC4), Small Intestine (MA-SC2), and Sympathetic (MA-AH7).

Supplementary Points: Spleen (MA-IC), Rectum (MA-H2), *Sān Jiāo* (MA-IC4), and Endocrine (MA-IC3).

THERAPEUTIC METHODS

Ear Acupuncture: Use all the primary points together with one or two supplementary points. Apply needle scratching and rotation; retain the needles 30 to 60 minutes and manipulate every 10 to 15 minutes. Treat once per day. Begin treatment on a single ear and change to the opposite ear every other day. One treatment course is five to ten days; allow two to three days between treatment courses.

Ear Acupressure: Use vaccaria seeds at all primary points together with supplementary points as needed. Press the seeds three to five times a day, two to three minutes each time. Begin treatment on a single ear and change to the opposite ear every five to seven days.

NOTES

- Ear acupuncture is also effective for patients with ulcerative colitis that flares up following a period of healing.
- In general, two or three additional treatment courses should be given for patients whose symptoms have disappeared, in order to strengthen the therapeutic effect.
- Fish, shrimp, and cold, raw, or irritating food should not be eaten during treatment.
- Ear acupuncture is used for the acute stage, while ear acupressure is more often used for the remission stage.
- Ear moxibustion can be added for those who experience frequent diarrhea.

Gastrointestinal Neurosis

TREATMENT PRESCRIPTION

Primary Points: Ear Shén Mén (MA-TF1), Sympathetic (MA-AH7), Heart (MA-IC), and Subcortex (MA-AT1).

Supplementary Points: Liver (MA-SC5), Adrenal Gland (MA-T), Occiput (MA-AT), Pancreas/Gallbladder (MA-SC6), Spleen (MA-IC), Stomach (MA-IC), Large Intestine (MA-SC4), and Small Intestine (MA-SC2).

THERAPEUTIC METHODS

Ear Acupressure: Use all the primary points together with a few supplementary points, according to the patient's condition. For example, add Spleen (MA-IC) and Stomach (MA-IC) for gastric neurosis; add Large Intestine (MA-SC4) and Small Intestine (MA-SC2) for intestinal neurosis. Press the vaccaria seeds three to five times a day, two to three minutes each time. Begin treatment on a single ear and change to the opposite ear every five to seven days.

Ear Acupuncture or Electroacupuncture: Treat sensitive points first, then the prescribed points. Retain the needles for 60 minutes (30 minutes for electroacupuncture) and manipulate every 10 to 15 minutes. Treat once per day. Begin treatment on a single ear and change to the opposite ear every other day. One treatment course is seven to ten days.

Constipation

TREATMENT PRESCRIPTION

Primary Points: Large Intestine (MA-SC4), Rectum (MA-H2), and Sympathetic (MA-AH7).

Supplementary Points: Spleen (MA-IC), Subcortex (MA-AT1), Lung (MA-IC1), Abdomen (MA-AH), and Small Intestine (MA-SC2).

THERAPEUTIC METHODS

Ear Acupuncture: Use all the primary points together with one or two supplementary points. For example, Spleen (MA-IC) and Lung (MA-IC1) treat vacuity pattern; Subcortex (MA-AT1) and Rectum (MA-H2) treat repletion pattern. Retain the needles for 30 to 60 minutes and manipulate every 10 to 15 minutes. Apply needle scratching and rotation using mild stimulation for vacuity pattern; rotate using stronger stimulation for repletion pattern. Treat once per day. Begin treatment on a single ear and change to the opposite ear every other day. One treatment course lasts five to seven days; allow two or three days between treatment courses.

Ear Acupressure: Affix vaccaria seeds at two or three primary points together with one or two supplementary points. Press the seeds three to five times per day, two to three minutes each time. Begin treatment on a single ear and change to the opposite ear every five to seven days.

Point Massage: The patient can do ear point massage independently.

Massage with Fingers: Press the triangular fossa and intertragic notch with the thumb and index finger in opposition. Particularly knead while pressing Large Intestine (MA-SC4) and Endocrine (MA-IC3) with a moderate force, alternately pressing forcefully and lifting. Knead while pressing each treated area or point 10 to 30 times, three times per day. Begin treatment on a single ear and change to the opposite ear every other day.

Pressing with a stick: Press the triangular fossa and intertragic notch points with a wooden, plastic, or glass stick until distention of the abdomen is induced. Repeat three to five times each day, two to three minutes each time. Treat alternate ears every other day.

NOTES

- The patient should schedule a regular time each day to have a bowel movement and press the prescribed points during defecation. The patient should also drink a glass of salty water (those with heart or kidney disease should drink plain warm water) every morning before breakfast. Roughage, fruits, chestnuts, sesame, and honey are recommended foods; acidic, hot, and irritating foods should not be eaten. Proper exercises may help reduce instances of constipation.

Diarrhea

TREATMENT PRESCRIPTION 1

Primary Points: Large Intestine (MA-SC4), Small Intestine (MA-SC2), Stomach (MA-IC), and Spleen (MA-IC).

Supplementary Points: Add Sympathetic (MA-AH7) and Ear Shén Mén (MA-TF1) for abdominal pain; add Ear Apex (MA-H6) for acute diarrhea; add Liver (MA-SC5), Kidney (MA-SC), and Endocrine (MA-IC3) for chronic diarrhea.

THERAPEUTIC METHODS

Ear Acupuncture: Use all the primary points together with supplementary points as needed. For acute diarrhea, treat both ears simultaneously; use strong stimulation by applying lifting and thrusting and needle rotation. Retain the needles 30 to 60 minutes and manipulate every 10 to 15 minutes. Treat once per day until diarrhea is stopped. For chronic diarrhea, each ear is treated on alternate days using mild stimulation by needle scratching and rotation. Retain the needles 30 minutes and manipulate the needles every 10 minutes. Treat once per day. One treatment course is five days; allow two or three days between treatment courses.

Ear Acupressure: Use three or four primary points together with supplementary points as needed. Treat both ears simultaneously for acute diarrhea. Press the vaccaria seeds three to five times each day, three to five minutes each time, or press until soreness and distention are induced. The same manipulation is to be done in one ear only for chronic diarrhea, changing to the opposite ear every five to seven days.

TREATMENT PRESCRIPTION 2

Primary Points: Large Intestine (MA-SC4), Ear Shén Mén (MA-TF1), Spleen (MA-IC), and Sympathetic (MA-AH7).

THERAPEUTIC METHOD

Medicine Injection: Commonly injected medications include Vitamin B_{12} with Vitamin B_1, berberine injection fluid, angelica injection fluid, and Novocain. For acute diarrhea, treat two times per day, using two to three prescribed points. Change to the opposite ear the next day, using two different points. If the treatment is not effective after four or five days, change to a different group of points. For chronic diarrhea, treat once per day at one or two of the points, changing points and to the opposite ear on alternate days. One treatment course is five to seven days; allow two or three days between treatment courses.

Biliary Ascariasis

TREATMENT PRESCRIPTION

Primary Points: Pancreas/Gallbladder (MA-SC6), Liver (MA-SC5), Ear Shén Mén (MA-TF1), and Sympathetic (MA-AH7).

Supplementary Points: Duodenum (MA-SC1), Root of Ear Vagus (MA-PS), and Stomach (MA-IC).

THERAPEUTIC METHOD

Ear Acupuncture: Use all the primary points together with supplementary points as needed. Treat both ears simultaneously, including applying lifting and thrusting and needle rotation until pain is relieved. Retain the needles 30 to 60 minutes and manipulate every 10 to 15 minutes.

NOTES

- Ear acupuncture is especially effective for treating biliary ascariasis. The stronger the stimulation, the better the therapeutic effect. Persistent strong stimulation can resolve tetany of the biliary tract and relax the sphincter of the biliary tract, which are beneficial to the bile and contribute to excreting worms.

Vomiting

TREATMENT PRESCRIPTION

Primary Points: Stomach (MA-IC), Ear Center (MA-H1), Subcortex (MA-AT1), Ear Shén Mén (MA-TF1), and Sympathetic (MA-AH7).

Supplementary Points: Occiput (MA-AT), Cervical Vertebrae (MA-AH8), Liver (MA-SC5), and Spleen (MA-IC).

Ear Acupuncture: Insert a needle at a sensitive spot near Stomach (MA-IC) and apply point joining to Ear Center (MA-H1); alternatively, insert a needle at a sensitive spot near Ear Center (MA-H1) and apply point joining to Stomach (MA-IC). Then needle Ear Shén Mén (MA-TF1), Subcortex (MA-AT1), and Sympathetic (MA-AH7) as well as one or two more supplementary points. For sudden onset of vomiting, treat both ears simultaneously, using strong stimulation, retaining the needles 30 to 60 minutes, and manipulating every 10 to 15 minutes. Treat one or two times per day. For chronic vomiting, start treatment on one ear, using mild manipulations such as needle scratching. Retain the needles 30 minutes and manipulate every 10 minutes. Change to the opposite ear every other day. One treatment course is seven to ten days; allow two to three days between treatment courses.

Ear Acupressure: Use three or four primary points together with supplementary points as needed. Both ears are used for a sudden attack of vomiting and one ear for chronic attacks, with a change to the opposite ear every five to seven days. Press the vaccaria seeds three to five times a day, two to three minutes each time, or until nausea and vomiting are relieved.

NOTES

- While ear acupuncture is effective for treating functional vomiting, projectile vomiting requires comprehensive medical care.

Hiccoughs

TREATMENT PRESCRIPTION 1

Primary Points: Diaphragm (Ear Center, MA-H1) (located on the helix root) and Stomach (MA-IC).

THERAPEUTIC METHOD

Electroacupuncture: Treat both ears simultaneously. Insert a needle at Stomach (MA-IC) in each ear and apply point joining to Diaphragm (Ear Center, MA-H1). Connect the inserted needles to an electroacupuncture apparatus, and select continuous wave type, increasing the current as much as the patient can tolerate until the hiccoughs are relieved. Continue the treatment for an additional 20 minutes to consolidate the therapeutic effect. In general, hiccoughs can be relieved with one treatment. Recurrent hiccoughs may also be treated with the same method.

TREATMENT PRESCRIPTION 2

Primary Points: Ear Center (MA-H1), Stomach (MA-IC), and Ear Shén Mén (MA-TF1).

Supplementary Points: Sympathetic (MA-AH7), Subcortex (MA-AT1), Kidney (MA-SC), and Spleen (MA-IC).

THERAPEUTIC METHODS

Ear Massage: Find the sensitive spot around Ear Center (MA-H1) with the index finger, and then press with the nail for three to five minutes until hiccoughs stop.

Needle Implantation: Select Ear Center (MA-H1) and Stomach (MA-IC). Support the auricle with one hand, while quickly inserting a filiform needle at Ear Center (MA-H1). Then slowly apply point joining to Stomach (MA-IC) while lifting and thrusting and using needle rotation until severe soreness, distention, and a sensation of heat are induced. Finally, retain the needle until the hiccoughs stop completely.

CASE STUDY: HICCOUGH

Zhu, a 70-year-old male, underwent surgery for hyperplasia of the prostate under extradural anesthesia of the spinal cord. Since the third day following surgery, he had suffered from severe, loud hiccoughs. The hiccoughs occurred two to three times per minute, and medication provided no relief.

Treatment Prescription: Ear Center (MA-H1), Stomach (MA-IC), Liver (MA-SC5), Cardiac (MA-IC7), Sympathetic (MA-AH7), Subcortex (MA-AT1), and Ear Shén Mén (MA-TF1).

Therapeutic Method: Needling both ears with 30 minutes of needle retention.

Treatment Results: The patient's hiccoughs started to decrease five minutes after treatment and completely stopped after 15 minutes. According to follow-up inquiries, the hiccoughs did not recur.

Comments: 1. Ear acupuncture has good therapeutic results for hiccoughs due to nerve reflex, but unsatisfactory results with hiccoughs due to CNS disorders.

2. Needles are used for the first treatment. Usually, hiccoughs can be resolved in 30 minutes. For recurrent onset, use ear seed acupressure. The patient should be instructed to press the seeds whenever he senses the hiccoughs are going to occur. Persist with treatment until hiccoughs have completely stopped for three days.

Esophagitis

TREATMENT PRESCRIPTION

Esophagus (MA-IC6), Cardiac (MA-IC7), Stomach (MA-IC), Ear Shén Mén (MA-TF1), and Duodenum (MA-SC1).

THERAPEUTIC METHODS

Ear Acupuncture: Select all the primary points and apply needle scratching and rotation. Retain the needles 30 to 60 minutes and manipulate every 10 to 15 minutes. Treat once per day. Begin treatment on a single ear and change to the opposite ear every other day. One treatment course is seven to ten days; allow two or three days between treatment courses.

Ear Acupressure: Use three to five of the prescribed points. Press the vaccaria seeds three to five times a day, two to three minutes each time. Begin treatment on a single ear and change to the opposite ear every five to seven days.

NOTES

- Ear acupuncture significantly improves all symptoms of esophagitis.
- Red spots with luster can be found at Esophagus (MA-IC6) and Stomach (MA-IC).

Cholecystitis

TREATMENT PRESCRIPTION

Primary Points: Liver (MA-SC5), Pancreas/Gallbladder (MA-SC6), Sympathetic (MA-AH7), and Ear Shén Mén (MA-TF1).

Supplementary Points: Ear Apex (MA-H6), Stomach (MA-IC), Large Intestine (MA-SC4), Small Intestine (MA-SC2), *Sān Jiāo* (MA-IC4), Endocrine (MA-IC3), and Duodenum (MA-SC1).

THERAPEUTIC METHODS

Ear Acupuncture: Use all the primary points together with one or two supplementary points; for example, add Ear Apex (MA-H6) for fever or Stomach (MA-IC) and Large Intestine (MA-SC4) for poor digestion and abdominal distention. Treat both ears simultaneously for acute cholecystitis. Treat once or twice per day; retain the needles 30 to 60 minutes and manipulate every 10 to 15 minutes using strong stimulation by applying needle rotation. For chronic cholecystitis, treat only one ear and treat once per day. Retain the needles 30 minutes and manipulate every 10 minutes using needle scratching and rotation. Change to the opposite ear every other day. Each treatment course lasts five to seven days; allow one or two days between treatment courses.

Ear Acupressure: Use three or four prescribed points. Press the vaccaria seeds three to five times per day, two to three minutes each time. Begin treatment on a single ear and change to the opposite ear every five to seven days.

Electroacupuncture: Insert needles into the main or supplementary points that are most sensitive. Connect these to an electroacupuncture apparatus at the sine wave setting. Treat once per day, five to ten minutes at each point. Begin treatment on a single ear and change to the opposite ear every other day. One treatment course is ten days.

NOTES

* The effectiveness of this therapy is closely related to appropriate determination of sensitive spots, intensity of stimulation, and manipulation of needles. In electroacupuncture, the patient should not feel pain nor experience any other impairment or side effect.

CASE STUDY: CHOLECYSTITIS

Xu, a 50-year-old male, reported that for more than two years he had dull pain in the gastric and hypochondriac regions on the right side as well as distending pain on the back of the right side. Greasy food intake and cold made these symptoms worse. He was treated for gastric disorder for several months with no result. The diagnosis from ultrasound B was "chronic cholecystitis."

Treatment Prescription: Liver (MA-SC5), Pancreas/Gallbladder (MA-SC6), Duodenum (MA-SC1), Biliary Duct *(Dǎn Guǎn),*[13] Stomach (MA-IC), Sympathetic (MA-AH7), and Adrenal Gland (MA-T).

Therapeutic Method: Seed acupressure was applied at all the above points, switching ears every three to five days. The patient was told to press the seeds three to five times per day during the treatment.

Treatment Results: The patient's dull gastric pain was relieved and the distending back pain went away after two treatments; also, his appetite was improving. All the symptoms were gone after six treatments.

Comment: Acute cholecystitis can also be treated with the above method to relieve gripping pain of the gallbladder, but other therapies should be added whenever the patient has a severe and/or complicated situation.

Nephritis

TREATMENT PRESCRIPTION

Primary Points: Bladder (MA-SC8), Kidney (MA-SC), Adrenal Gland (MA-T), Sympathetic (MA-AH7), and *Sān Jiāo* (MA-IC4).

Supplementary Points: Occiput (MA-AT), Ear Shén Mén (MA-TF1), Endocrine (MA-IC3), Spleen (MA-IC), Urethra (MA-H3), Groove of Posterior Surface (MA-PS), and Lung (MA-IC1).

THERAPEUTIC METHODS

Ear Acupuncture: Select two or three primary points together with one or two supplementary points according to the patient's specific condition. For example, add Lung (MA-IC1) and Urethra (MA-H3) for acute nephritis; add Spleen (MA-IC) and Endocrine (MA-IC3) for chronic nephritis; add Ear Shén Mén (MA-TF1) and Groove of Posterior Surface (MA-PS) for hypertension. Retain the needles 30 minutes and manipulate every 10 minutes using needle scratching and rotation. Treat once per day. Begin treatment on a single ear and change to the opposite ear every other day. One treatment course is seven to ten days.

Ear Acupressure: Select three to five primary points and supplementary points as needed. Affix vaccaria seeds and press them three to five times each day, two to three minutes each time. Begin treatment on a single ear and change to the opposite ear every five to seven days.

---

[13] This is an empirical point located midway between Pancreas/Gallbladder (MA-SC6) and Duodenum (MA-SC1). (See Figure 2.13, page 42.)

TREATMENT PRESCRIPTION 2

Primary Point: Kidney (MA-SC).

THERAPEUTIC METHOD

Ear Acupuncture: Needle at the sensitive spot around Kidney (MA-SC) using needle scratching and rotation; retain the inserted needle four to six hours and manipulate every 30 minutes. One treatment course lasts seven days.

Pyelonephritis

TREATMENT PRESCRIPTION

Primary Points: Kidney (MA-SC), *Sān Jiāo* (MA-IC4), and Bladder (MA-SC8).

Supplementary Points: Ear Apex (MA-H6), Spleen (MA-IC), Lung (MA-IC1), Sympathetic (MA-AH7), and Adrenal Gland (MA-T).

THERAPEUTIC METHODS

Ear Acupuncture: Select two or three primary points together with one or two supplementary points; for example, add Ear Apex (MA-H6) (bloodletting) and Lung (MA-IC1) for acute pyelonephritis with fever; add Spleen (MA-IC) and Adrenal Gland (MA-T) for chronic pyelonephritis. Treat both ears simultaneously for acute pyelonephritis. Retain the needles 60 minutes and manipulate every 15 minutes. One treatment course is five to seven days. For chronic cases, retain the needles 30 minutes and manipulate every 10 minutes. Begin treatment on a single ear and change to the opposite ear every other day. Each treatment course is seven to ten days.

Ear Acupressure: Select all the primary points together with supplementary points as needed. Affix vaccaria seeds and press them three to five times, two to three minutes each time. Begin treatment on a single ear and change to the opposite ear every five to seven days.

NOTES

- Ear acupuncture is effective for treating pyelonephritis regardless of whether it is acute or chronic.
- A better therapeutic effect is achieved by giving a few extra treatments after all symptoms are gone.
- Low-salt food and proper rest are needed in combination with ear acupuncture to treat this disorder.

Chyluria (Hazy Urine)

TREATMENT PRESCRIPTION 1

Primary Points: Kidney (MA-SC), Bladder (MA-SC8), Subcortex (MA-AT1), and Ear Shén Mén (MA-TF1).

THERAPEUTIC METHOD

Medicine Injection: A mixture totaling 0.1 ml of vitamins B_1 and B_{12} is used for each point. Begin treatment on a single ear and change to the opposite ear every other day. One treatment course is seven days; allow two to three days between treatment courses.

TREATMENT PRESCRIPTION 2

Primary Points: Kidney (MA-SC), Endocrine (MA-IC3), and Bladder (MA-SC8).

Supplementary Points: *Sān Jiāo* (MA-IC4), Urethra (MA-H3), Subcortex (MA-AT1), and Ear Shén Mén (MA-TF1).

THERAPEUTIC METHOD

Ear Acupuncture: Use all the primary points together with one or two supplementary points. Retain the needles 30 to 60 minutes and manipulate every 10 to 15 minutes using needle rotation. Begin treatment on a single ear and change to the opposite ear every other day. One treatment course is seven to ten days; allow two or three days between treatment courses.

NOTES

- Ear acupuncture is not recommended for treating chyluria resulting from cancer. A better therapeutic effect can be achieved with Western medicinal treatments such as Hetrazan.

Excess Residual Urine

TREATMENT PRESCRIPTION

Primary Points: Ureter (MA-SC7), Kidney (MA-SC), and Bladder (MA-SC8).

Supplementary Points: Sympathetic (MA-AH7), Subcortex (MA-AT1), and Ear Shén Mén (MA-TF1).

THERAPEUTIC METHOD

Ear Acupressure: Select all primary points together with one or two supplementary points. Affix vaccaria seeds and press them three to five times a day, two to three minutes each time. Begin treatment on a single ear and change to the opposite ear every five to seven days.

NOTES

*   Ear acupuncture is very effective for treating excess residual urine. Of 34 patients with this condition, 16 were completely healed, five were greatly improved, and only three were not helped at all by this treatment.

Urinary Incontinence

TREATMENT PRESCRIPTION 1

Primary Points: Bladder (MA-SC8), Ear Shén Mén (MA-TF1), Subcortex (MA-AT1), and Kidney (MA-SC).

THERAPEUTIC METHODS

Ear Acupuncture: Select all the primary points. Treat both ears simultaneously. Retain the needles for 30 to 60 minutes and manipulate every 10 to 15 minutes. Treat once per day. In general, three to five treatments can cure this disorder. Treat three times more on an every-other-day basis to consolidate the therapeutic effect.

Ear Acupressure: Select all the primary points. Affix vaccaria seeds and press them three to five times a day, one to three minutes each time. Begin treatment on a single ear and change to the opposite ear every five to seven days.

TREATMENT PRESCRIPTION 2

Primary Points: Kidney (MA-SC), and Bladder (MA-SC8).

THERAPEUTIC METHOD

Medicine Injection: Fix the auricle with one hand, then inject 0.2 ml of thiamine into the prescribed points one by one, pressing each point after withdrawing the syringe. Begin treatment on a single ear and change to the opposite ear every other day. One treatment course is five to seven days; allow two to three days between treatment courses.

Frequent Urination

TREATMENT PRESCRIPTION

Primary Points: Bladder (MA-SC8), Kidney (MA-SC), and Subcortex (MA-AT1).

Supplementary Points: Central Rim (MA-AT), Spleen (MA-IC), Sympathetic (MA-AH7), Ear Shén Mén (MA-TF1), *Sān Jiāo* (MA-IC4), Adrenal Gland (MA-T), and Endocrine (MA-IC3).

THERAPEUTIC METHODS

Ear Acupuncture: Use all the primary points together with one or two supplementary points; for example, add Spleen (MA-IC), Endocrine (MA-IC3), and Adrenal Gland (MA-T) for kidney-bladder vacuity cold; add *Sān Jiāo* (MA-IC4), Sympathetic (MA-AH7), and Ear Shén Mén (MA-TF1) for damp-heat pouring downward. Retain the needles 30 to 60 minutes and manipulate every 10 to 15 minutes. Begin treatment on a single ear and change to the opposite ear every five to seven days (one treatment course); allow one to three days between treatment courses.

Ear Acupressure: Use all the primary points together with supplementary points as needed. Press the vaccaria seeds three to five times per day, one to three minutes each time. Begin treatment on a single ear and change to the opposite ear every five to seven days.

CASE STUDY: FREQUENT URINATION

Guo, a 9-year-old girl, reported that she had frequent urination for three months with urination every 10 to 15 minutes. When she was nervous the symptom was worse. A physical examination revealed no clear cause of this problem. The diagnosis was "nervous frequent urination."

Treatment Prescription: Kidney (MA-SC), Bladder (MA-SC8), Ear Center (MA-H1), Central Rim (MA-AT), Subcortex (MA-AT1), and Sympathetic (MA-AH7).

Therapeutic Method: Seed acupressure was used on one ear at a time, switching ears twice a week.

Treatment Results: The frequency of urination was significantly decreased after two treatments. Urination returned to normal after six treatments (with urination every three to four hours). For enhancing the therapeutic results, a total of eight treatments were given. No other therapy was applied during the ear acupuncture treatments.

Retention of Urine

TREATMENT PRESCRIPTION

Primary Points: Kidney (MA-SC), Bladder (MA-SC8), and Subcortex (MA-AT1).

Supplementary Points: Ureter (MA-SC7), *Sān Jiāo* (MA-IC4), Ear Shén Mén (MA-TF1), and Urethra (MA-H3).

THERAPEUTIC METHODS

Electroacupuncture: Use all the primary points together with one or two supplementary points; for example, add *Sān Jiāo* (MA-IC4) and

Ureter (MA-SC7) for functional reflex retention of urine; add Ear Shén Mén (MA-TF1) for retention of urine due to nerve damage or nerve condition. Insert needles into the selected points, then connect the needles to an electroacupuncture apparatus using continuous wave setting; retain for 30 minutes. Begin treatment on a single ear and change to the opposite ear every other day. One treatment course is five to seven days.

Ear Acupressure: Select the same points as above. Affix vaccaria seeds and press them three to five times a day, one to three minutes each time. Begin treatment on a single ear and change to the opposite ear every five to seven days.

NOTES

- Ear acupuncture is significantly effective for treating nervous and reflex retention of urine. Urination can occur after just one treatment in some cases.
- There is no reliable therapeutic effect for treating mechanical retention of urine.

Erectile Dysfunction (Impotence)

TREATMENT PRESCRIPTION

Primary Points: Kidney (MA-SC), Subcortex (MA-AT1), and External Genitals (MA-H4).

Supplementary Points: Ear Shén Mén (MA-TF1), Endocrine (MA-IC3), Spleen (MA-IC), Stomach (MA-IC), Sympathetic (MA-AH7), and Heart (MA-IC).

THERAPEUTIC METHODS

Ear Acupuncture: Use all the primary points together with one or two supplementary points; for example, add Ear Shén Mén (MA-TF1) for insomnia and forgetfulness; add Stomach (MA-IC) and Spleen (MA-IC) for poor appetite. Retain the needles 30 to 60 minutes and manipulate every 10 to 15 minutes using needle scratching and rotation. Begin treatment on a single ear and change to the opposite ear every other day. One treatment course is seven to ten days; allow one to three days between treatment courses.

Ear Acupressure: Use all the primary points together with supplementary points as needed. Press the vaccaria seeds three to five times per day, one to three minutes each time. Begin treatment on a single ear and change to the opposite ear every five to seven days.

CASE STUDY: IMPOTENCE

Lu, a 29-year-old male, reported that his penis was unable to become erect. This started with fright during sex. A physical examination revealed no explanation for this problem. The diagnosis was "dysfunctional impotence."

Treatment Prescription: Internal Reproductive Organs (MA-TF), External Genitals (MA-H4), Testicle (MA-AT), Liver (MA-SC5), Heart (MA-IC), Adrenal Gland (MA-T), Subcortex (MA-AT1), and Central Rim (MA-AT).

Therapeutic Method: Seed acupressure was used on one ear at a time, switching ears twice a week. The patient was told to press the seeds three to five times per day during the treatment.

Treatment Results: The patient was able to have sex on the same day as the initial day of treatment. To enhance the therapeutic results, a total of four treatments were given.

Comments: 1. Although there are many causes of impotence, ear acupuncture is only effective for dysfunctional impotence.

2. Psychological treatment should also be used in order to ease the patient's mental pressure and to build the patient's confidence in a successful therapeutic outcome from ear acupuncture.

Seminal Emission

TREATMENT PRESCRIPTION

Primary Points: Kidney (MA-SC), Heart (MA-IC), Subcortex (MA-AT1), and Ear Shén Mén (MA-TF1).

Supplementary Points: Adrenal Gland (MA-T), *Sān Jiāo* (MA-IC4), Liver (MA-SC5), Spleen (MA-IC), Endocrine (MA-IC3), and Internal Reproductive Organs (MA-TF).

THERAPEUTIC METHODS

Ear Acupuncture: Select one to three primary points together with one or two supplementary points. Manipulate by needle scratching and rotation. Retain the needles 30 minutes and manipulate every 10 minutes. Begin treatment on a single ear and change to the opposite ear every five to seven days (one treatment course).

Ear Acupressure: Select the same points as above. Affix vaccaria seeds and press them three times per day, three minutes each time. Begin treatment on a single ear and change to the opposite ear every five to seven days.

CASE STUDY: SEMINAL EMISSION

Leng, a 40-year-old male, had nocturnal seminal emission two to three
times per week for the last three years, along with dizziness, soreness and weakness of the lumbar region, listlessness, and lassitude. A physical examination revealed no explanation for this
problem. The diagnosis was "seminal emission."

Treatment Prescription: Kidney (MA-SC), Heart (MA-IC), Liver (MA-
SC5), Subcortex (MA-AT1), Occiput (MA-AT), and Anterior Ear
Lobe (MA-L).

Therapeutic Method: Seed acupressure for all the above points,
switching ears twice every week. The patient was told to press the
seeds three to five times per day during the treatment.

Treatment Results: Nocturnal seminal emission only occurred once
after two treatments and once again after one month of treatment.
All the associated symptoms were relieved.

Comments: 1. Treatment of seminal emission with ear acupuncture
has consistently good results when seminal emission is a dysfunctional disorder.

2. For better and faster therapeutic effects, psychological
therapy should be added to enhance the patient's confidence a
positive oucome.

Prostatitis

TREATMENT PRESCRIPTION

Primary Points: Internal Reproductive Organs (MA-TF), Bladder (MA-SC8), Endocrine (MA-IC3), and Ear Shén Mén (MA-TF1).

Supplementary Points: Adrenal Gland (MA-T), Pelvis (MA-TF),
Ureter (MA-SC7), Ear Apex (MA-H6), Helix 1-6 (MA-H 1-6), External
Genitals (MA-H4), and Subcortex (MA-AT1).

THERAPEUTIC METHODS

Ear Acupuncture: Select one to three primary points together with
one or two supplementary points; for example, add Ear Apex (MA-H6)
(bloodletting) and Helix 1-6 (MA-H 1-6) for acute prostatitis; add External
Genitals (MA-H4) for painful perineum; add Subcortex (MA-AT1) and
Adrenal Gland (MA-T) for sexual hypoesthesia. For acute prostatitis, use
strong stimulation by applying lifting and thrusting and needle rotation,
treating both ears simultaneously. Retain the needles 60 minutes and manipulate every 15 minutes. Treat once per day. For chronic prostatitis,
needle scratching and rotation are used. Retain the needles 30 minutes and
manipulate every 10 minutes. Begin treatment on a single ear and change

to the opposite ear every five to seven days (one treatment course); allow one to three days between treatment courses.

Ear Acupressure: Select the same points as above. Press the vaccaria seeds three to five times per day, one to three minutes each time. Begin treatment on a single ear and change to the opposite ear every five to seven days.

NOTES

- Ear acupuncture is very effective in treating prostatitis.
- White spots with changes of luster or pitting or prominences can be found at Endocrine (MA-IC3) or Bladder (MA-SC8) in patients with prostatitis.

CASE STUDY: PROSTATITIS

Cao, a 26-year-old male, reported that for one month he had discomfort around the perineal region as well as frequent urination, dizziness, soreness of the lumbar region, listlessness and lassitude, and insomnia. Prostate test showed swelling and softening; ESP results: white, WBC (+), 60% lecithin, no micro-organism growth with cultivation. The diagnosis was "chronic non-infectious prostatitis."

Treatment Prescription: Internal Reproductive Organs (MA-TF), Kidney (MA-SC), Prostate/Angle of Superior Concha (MA-SC), Testicle (MA-AT), Adrenal Gland (MA-T), Subcortex (MA-AT1), and Anterior Ear Lobe (MA-L).

Therapeutic Method: Seed acupressure was applied to all the above points, switching ears twice a week. The patient was told to press the seeds three to five times per day during the treatment.

Treatment Results: All the symptoms started to improve after four treatments, particularly insomnia. All the symptoms were gone after eight treatments. Another four treatments were given to enhance the therapeutic results.

Comment: Ear acupuncture is more effective for non-infectious prostatitis.

Diabetes

TREATMENT PRESCRIPTION 1

Right Ear Points: Endocrine (MA-IC3), Lung (MA-IC1), Stomach (MA-IC), Pancreas/Gallbladder (MA-SC6), Central Rim (MA-AT), and Adrenal Gland (MA-T).

Left Ear Points: Endocrine (MA-IC3), Lung (MA-IC1), Spleen (MA-IC), Kidney (MA-SC), *Sān Jiāo* (MA-IC4), and Apex of Antitragus (MA-AT).

THERAPEUTIC METHODS

Ear Acupuncture: Use all the points in one ear for one treatment. Insert needles slowly while applying needle scratching and rotation until distention and a dragging feeling are induced. Retain the needles 60 minutes and manipulate every 15 minutes. Treat once per day. Begin treatment on a single ear and change to the opposite ear every other day. One treatment course is 30 days.

TREATMENT PRESCRIPTION 2

Primary Points: Pancreas/Gallbladder (MA-SC6), Endocrine (MA-IC3).

Supplementary Points: Kidney (MA-SC), *Sān Jiāo* (MA-IC4), Root of Ear Vagus (MA-PS), Ear Shén Mén (MA-TF1), Heart (MA-IC), Liver (MA-SC5), Spleen (MA-IC), Stomach (MA-IC), and Bladder (MA-SC8).

THERAPEUTIC METHODS

Ear Acupressure: Use all the primary points together with one or two supplementary points. For example, add Heart (MA-IC) and Ear Shén Mén (MA-TF1) for upper dispersion; add Stomach (MA-IC) and Liver (MA-SC5) for center dispersion; add Liver (MA-SC5), Kidney (MA-SC), and Bladder (MA-SC8) for lower dispersion. Press the vaccaria seeds three to five times per day, one to three minutes each time. Begin treatment on a single ear and change to the opposite ear every five to seven days.

Medicine Injection: This method is for patients with low levels of insulin. Use 50u of insulin dissolved in 1 ml 0.9% normal saline. Select three to five of the prescribed points, and inject 0.1–0.2 ml at each point once every other day. Begin with a single ear and change to the opposite ear every other session.

NOTES

• Ear acupuncture can significantly reduce both blood sugar and urine sugar levels when applied in combination with a proper diet.

Hyperthyroidism

TREATMENT PRESCRIPTION

Primary Points: Endocrine (MA-IC3), Subcortex (MA-AT1), and Ear Shén Mén (MA-TF1).

Supplementary Points: Heart (MA-IC), Liver (MA-SC5), Lung (MA-IC1), Kidney (MA-SC), Stomach (MA-IC), Sympathetic (MA-AH7), Adrenal Gland (MA-T), and Root of Ear Vagus (MA-PS).

THERAPEUTIC METHODS

Ear Acupuncture: Select one to three primary points together with one or two supplementary points. Add needle scratching and rotation manipulations. Retain the needles 30 minutes and manipulate every 10 minutes. Treat once per day. Begin treatment on a single ear and change to the opposite ear every other day. One treatment course is seven to ten days; allow one to three days between treatment courses.

Ear Acupressure: Select the same points as above. Affix vaccaria seeds and press them three to five times per day, one to three minutes each time. Begin treatment on a single ear and change to the opposite ear every five to seven days.

Headache

TREATMENT PRESCRIPTION

Primary Points: Ear Shén Mén (MA-TF1), Subcortex (MA-AT1), Forehead (MA-AT), Occiput (MA-AT), and Temple (MA-AT).

Supplementary Points: Ear Apex (MA-H6), Heart (MA-IC), Liver (MA-SC5), Helix 1-6 (MA-H 1-6), Kidney (MA-SC), Endocrine (MA-IC3), Upper Ear Root (MA-PS), Groove of Posterior Surface (MA-PS), Cheek (MA-L), Eye (MA-L1), Internal Nose (MA-T), Cervical Vertebrae (MA-AH8), and Root of Ear Vagus (MA-PS).

THERAPEUTIC METHODS

Ear Acupuncture: Use all the primary points together with two or three supplementary points. For example, add Ear Apex (MA-H6) and Helix 1-6 (MA-H 1-6) (bloodletting) for headache with fever; add Forehead (MA-AT), Kidney (MA-SC), and Groove of Posterior Surface (MA-PS) (bloodletting) for headache seen in hypertension. For severe headaches, treat both ears simultaneously, using strong stimulation by applying lifting and thrusting and needle rotation. Retain the needles one to two hours, and manipulate every 15 to 30 minutes. Treat once or twice each day. Continue treatments until headaches are greatly improved or even completely cured. In general, severe headaches are greatly improved after three to five treatments. If not, discontinue ear acupuncture and change to another therapy, such as body acupuncture. For mild headaches, begin treatment on a single ear and change to the opposite ear every other day. Retain the needles 30 minutes and manipulate every 10 minutes, using needle scratching and rotation. Treat once per day. One treatment course lasts five to seven days; allow two or three days between treatment courses.

Ear Acupressure: Use three to five primary points together with supplementary points as needed. Press the vaccaria seeds three to five times per day, two to three minutes each time. Begin treatment on a single ear and change to the opposite ear every five to seven days.

Magnet Therapy: Select a pair of prescribed points that includes one point on the posterior surface of the auricle and the other on the anterior surface according to the patient's condition. Affix 1000 to 2000G magnetic beads at the selected points, with the poles of the magnets in opposition. Press the beads three times per day, two to three minutes each time. Begin treatment on a single ear and change to the opposite ear every third day.

CASE STUDY: MIGRAINE

Hu, a 40-year-old female, had suffered for many years from severe headache during her menstrual period, sometimes accompanied with vomiting. The headaches lasted one to two days. The patient had a flushed face, and her blood pressure was in the normal range. The diagnosis was "migraine."

Treatment Prescription: Ear Apex (MA-H6), Temple (MA-AT), Pancreas/Gallbladder (MA-SC6), Liver (MA-SC5), Sympathetic (MA-AH7), Ear Shén Mén (MA-TF1), Subcortex (MA-AT1), and Endocrine (MA-IC3).

Therapeutic Method: Bleeding at Ear Apex (MA-H6); seed acupressure for all other points with strong stimulation by kneading while pressing. Both ears were treated simultaneously and the seeds were changed twice a week. The patient was told to press the seeds three to five times per day during the treatment.

Treatment Results: The headache was remarkably relieved after 10 minutes' treatment, and the pain was gone after 30 minutes. The seeds were left on the points for the next three days to enhance the therapeutic effect. Subsequently, the patient was treated once a month during every period, and her headache was significantly controlled.

Comments: 1. Headache has many caues; ear acupuncture is most effective for dysfunctional headache.

2. The therapeutic effect of ear acupuncture on migraine is effective and reliable, but complete relief needs a long treatment course.

Anxiety Neurosis

TREATMENT PRESCRIPTION 1

Primary Points: Ear Shén Mén (MA-TF1), Heart (MA-IC), and Subcortex (MA-AT1).

Supplementary Points: Kidney (MA-SC), Stomach (MA-IC), Liver (MA-SC5), and Endocrine (MA-IC3).

THERAPEUTIC METHODS

Ear Acupuncture: Use all the primary points together with one or two supplementary points. For example, add Kidney (MA-SC) for palpitations; add Liver (MA-SC5) for irritability; add Endocrine (MA-IC3) for irregular menstrual cycle. Begin treatment on a single ear and change to the opposite ear every other day, using needle scratching and rotation. Retain the needles 30 minutes and manipulate every 10 minutes. Treat once per day; one treatment course is seven to ten days.

Ear Acupressure: Select the same points as above. Press the seeds three to five times per day, two to three minutes each time. Begin treatment on a single ear and change to the opposite ear every five to seven days.

Magnet Therapy: Use 500 to 1000G magnetic beads. Select three or four points and treat one time per week. Begin treatment on a single ear and change to the opposite ear every session.

CASE STUDY: ANXIETY NEUROSIS

Zhu, a 20-year-old male, reported that for two years he had severe insomnia, listlessness, lassitude, dizziness, and forgetfulness. To achieve sleep he had depended on insomnia medication for a long time. A physical examination revealed no explanation for this problem. The diagnosis was "acute anxiety neurosis (*shén jīng shuāi ruò*)."

Treatment Prescription: Heart (MA-IC), Kidney (MA-SC), Liver (MA-SC5), Subcortex (MA-AT1), Ear Shén Mén (MA-TF1), Occiput (MA-AT), and Anterior Ear Lobe (MA-L).

Therapeutic Method: Seed acupressure was used for all the above points, switching ears twice a week. The patient was told to press the seeds three to five times per day during the treatment.

Treatment Results: The patient slept better on the night of the first treatment, and his sleep returned to normal after six treatments while other symptoms were greatly improved. All the symptoms were gone after eight treatments.

Comment: Communicating with patients who suffer from mental diseases in order to relieve mental depression is a very important enhancement to ear acupuncture therapy.

Hysteria

TREATMENT PRESCRIPTION

Primary Points: Heart (MA-IC), Subcortex (MA-AT1), and Ear Shén Mén (MA-TF1).

Supplementary Points: Occiput (MA-AT), Liver (MA-SC5), Endocrine (MA-IC3), and other points corresponding to affected organ or area.[14]

THERAPEUTIC METHODS

Ear Acupuncture: Use all the primary points together with one or two supplementary points. For example, add Liver (MA-SC5) for moodiness; add Endocrine (MA-IC3), Occiput (MA-AT), Stomach (MA-IC), and Large Intestine (MA-SC4) for dysfunction of internal organs or the autonomic nervous system; add Occiput (MA-AT) and Lumbosacral Vertebrae (MA-AH) for paralysis. Treat both ears simultaneously in the acute stage, using lifting and thrusting and needle scratching; treatments should continue until manifestations disappear. During remission, treat one ear each day, alternating ears every other day, and use needle scratching and rotation. Retain the needles 30 minutes and manipulate every 10 minutes. One treatment course is five to seven days; allow two or three days between treatment courses.

Ear Acupressure: Select the same points as above. Affix vaccaria seeds and press them three to five times per day, two to three minutes each time. Begin treatment on a single ear and change to the opposite ear every five to seven days.

NOTES

- Hysteria is a psychological disorder, so mental therapy is needed in conjunction with ear acupuncture.

CASE STUDY: HYSTERIA

Qian, a 34-year-old female, had experienced an angry outburst and had subsequently suffered for 10 days from inability to stand and walk. Prior to the incident she had normal health. A nervous system examination revealed no explanation for this problem. The diagnosis was "hysteria."

Treatment Prescription: Liver (MA-SC5), Pancreas/Gallbladder (MA-SC6), Heart (MA-IC), Subcortex (MA-AT1), Sympathetic (MA-AH7), and Ear Shén Mén (MA-TF1).

Therapeutic Method: Simultaneously needle all the above points on both ears with strong stimulation.

---

[14] *Editor's Note:* When "corresponding points" are indicated, it simply means that the disease under discussion may occur at different locations around the body and the practitioner must pick points for the affected part, as well as the suggested systemic points for the problem.

Treatment Results: After 10 minutes of needling the patient was able to stand up with support. The needles were retained for 30 minutes and movement in both legs returned to normal. She walked home unassisted.

Comments: 1. Organic changes should be ruled out before choosing ear acupuncture therapy for hysterical diseases.

2. For patients with hysteria ear acupuncture should be combined with psychological therapy.

Epilepsy

TREATMENT PRESCRIPTION

Primary Points: Ear Shén Mén (MA-TF1), Heart (MA-IC), Central Rim (MA-AT), and Liver (MA-SC5).

Supplementary Points: Stomach (MA-IC), Spleen (MA-IC), Pancreas/Gallbladder (MA-SC6), Kidney (MA-SC), Subcortex (MA-AT1), and Occiput (MA-AT).

THERAPEUTIC METHODS

Ear Acupuncture: Use all the primary points together with one or two supplementary points. Treat both ears simultaneously for an acute attack, using strong stimulation by applying lifting and thrusting and needle rotation. Continue manipulation until all symptoms are resolved. During remission, treat one ear each day, alternating ears every other day. Retain the needles 30 to 60 minutes and manipulate every 10 to 15 minutes. One treatment course is seven to ten days.

Magnet Therapy: Select the same points as above. Press the beads three to five times a day, two to three minutes each time. Begin treatment on a single ear and change to the opposite ear every five to seven days.

NOTES

• Ear acupuncture is certainly effective in treating epilepsy. Younger patients with a more recent onset of epilepsy respond best to this therapy.

Mental Disturbance

TREATMENT PRESCRIPTION 1

Primary Points: Ear Shén Mén (MA-TF1).

THERAPEUTIC METHOD

Medicine Injection: Inject the point with 0.1–0.2 ml of compound vitamins one time per day for five to seven days. Begin treatment on a single ear and change to the opposite ear every other day.

TREATMENT PRESCRIPTION 2

Primary Points: Ear Shén Mén (MA-TF1), Heart (MA-IC), Liver (MA-SC5), and Subcortex (MA-AT1).

Supplementary Points: Stomach (MA-IC), Kidney (MA-SC), Adrenal Gland (MA-T), Endocrine (MA-IC3), Occiput (MA-AT), and Temple (MA-AT).

THERAPEUTIC METHOD

Needle Implantation: Select two primary points together with one or two supplementary points. Implant the needles at the selected points, then press the needles three to five times per day, two to three minutes each time. Begin treatment on a single ear and change to the opposite ear every five to seven days.

Competition Anxiety

TREATMENT PRESCRIPTION 1

Primary Points: Ear Shén Mén (MA-TF1) and Subcortex (MA-AT1).

Supplementary Points: Liver (MA-SC5), Heart (MA-IC), Sympathetic (MA-AH7), Occiput (MA-AT), Stomach (MA-IC), Endocrine (MA-IC3), and Adrenal Gland (MA-T).

THERAPEUTIC METHOD

Ear Acupressure: Use vitex seeds. Both primary points are used together with one or two supplementary points according to the patient's specific condition. For example, add Heart (MA-IC) and Kidney (MA-SC) for insomnia; add Stomach (MA-IC) for nausea and vomiting; add Endocrine (MA-IC3) for irregular menstrual cycle. Beginning two to three days before the test or competition, have the patient press the seeds three to five times a day, two to three minutes each time. Continue the treatment for a day or two after the examination.

TREATMENT PRESCRIPTION 2

Primary Points: Sensitive points on the auricle.

THERAPEUTIC METHOD

Needle Implantation: Sensitive points can be detected with a stimulator. Select two or three points, implant needles into the points, and press the needles three to five times per day, two to three minutes each time. Begin treatment on a single ear and change to the opposite ear every five to seven days, as necessary.

CASE STUDY: COMPETITION ANXIETY

CASE STUDY: COMPETITION ANXIETY

Gu, a 17-year-old female, reported that she recently had severe nervousness prior to participating in a national contest. Her symptoms included insomnia, palpitations, poor appetite, listlessness, and lassitude. She had always been nervous before or during any type of performance or competition. Her blood pressure was 125/80 mm Hg. Her heartbeat was 96/min. The diagnosis was "performance anxiety."

Treatment Prescription: Heart (MA-IC), Kidney (MA-SC), Liver (MA-SC5), Sympathetic (MA-AH7), Subcortex (MA-AT1), and Ear Shén Mén (MA-TF1).

Therapeutic Method: Seed acupressure was applied to all the points, switching ears twice a week. The patient was told to press the seeds three to five times per day during the treatment.

Treatment Results: All the above symptoms were gone after two treatments.

Comment: Ear acupuncture has a satisfactory therapeutic result for this disorder.

Rheumatism and Rheumatoid Arthritis

TREATMENT PRESCRIPTION

Primary Points: Ear Shén Mén (MA-TF1), Sympathetic (MA-AH7), Adrenal Gland (MA-T), and Subcortex (MA-AT1).

Supplementary Points: Bladder (MA-SC8), Spleen (MA-IC), Kidney (MA-SC), Liver (MA-SC5), and ear points corresponding to the affected areas.

THERAPEUTIC METHODS

Ear Acupuncture: Select two or three primary points together with one or two supplementary points. Retain the needles 30 to 60 minutes and manipulate every 10 to 15 minutes, using needle scratching and rotation. Treat once per day. Begin treatment on a single ear and change to the opposite ear every other day. One treatment course is seven to ten days; allow two or three days between treatment courses.

Ear Acupressure: Select the same points as above. Press the seeds three to five times a day, two to three minutes each time. Begin treatment on a single ear and change to the opposite ear every five to seven days.

Gout

TREATMENT PRESCRIPTION

Primary Points: Ear Shén Mén (MA-TF1), Endocrine (MA-IC3), and Subcortex (MA-AT1).

Supplementary Points: Kidney (MA-SC), Heart (MA-IC), Liver (MA-SC5), Spleen (MA-IC), and corresponding points.

THERAPEUTIC METHODS

Ear Acupuncture: Select two or three primary points together with one or two supplementary points. Treat both ears simultaneously in the acute stage, using strong stimulation by applying lifting and thrusting and needle rotation; retain the needles 30 to 60 minutes and manipulate every 10 to 15 minutes. Treat once per day. During periods of remission, use needle scratching and rotation. Continue to treat once per day, treating each ear on the alternate day. One treatment course is seven to ten days; allow two or three days between treatment courses.

Ear Acupressure: Select the same points as above. Press the seeds three to five times per day, two to three minutes each time. Begin treatment on a single ear and change to the opposite ear every five to seven days.

Anemia

TREATMENT PRESCRIPTION

Primary Points: Liver (MA-SC5), Heart (MA-IC), and Stomach (MA-IC).

Supplementary Points: Kidney (MA-SC), Spleen (MA-IC), *Sān Jiāo* (MA-IC4), and Endocrine (MA-IC3).

THERAPEUTIC METHODS

Ear Acupuncture: Use all the primary points together with one or two supplementary points. Retain the needles 30 minutes and manipulate every 10 minutes, using needle scratching or rotation. Treat once per day. Begin treatment on a single ear and change to the opposite ear every other day. One treatment course is seven to ten days; allow two or three days between treatment courses.

Ear Acupressure: Select the same points as above. Affix vaccaria seeds and press them three to five times per day, two to three minutes each time. Begin treatment on a single ear and change to the opposite ear every five to seven days.

NOTES

• Ear acupuncture treats anemia by increasing hemoglobin and improving all symptoms.

- Aplastic anemia should be treated with ear acupuncture in combination with other therapies.

Leukopenia

TREATMENT PRESCRIPTION 1

Primary Points: Liver (MA-SC5), Spleen (MA-IC), Kidney (MA-SC), and Endocrine (MA-IC3).

Supplementary Points: Adrenal Gland (MA-T), Ear Shén Mén (MA-TF1), Heart (MA-IC), Stomach (MA-IC), and Sympathetic (MA-AH7).

THERAPEUTIC METHODS

Ear Acupuncture: Select two or three primary points together with one or two supplementary points. Retain the needles 30 to 60 minutes and manipulate every 10 to 15 minutes, using needle scratching or rotation. Treat once per day. Begin treatment on a single ear and change to the opposite ear every other day. One treatment course is ten days.

Ear Acupressure: Select the same points as above. Press the seeds three to five times a day, two to three minutes each time. Begin treatment on a single ear and change to the opposite ear every five to seven days.

TREATMENT PRESCRIPTION 2

Primary Points: Ear Shén Mén (MA-TF1) and Kidney (MA-SC).

THERAPEUTIC METHOD

Moxibustion: Treat both points with stick incense for 20 to 30 minutes at each point per day. Begin treatment on a single ear and change to the opposite ear every other day. One treatment course is ten days; allow two to three days between treatment courses.

Thrombocytopenic Purpura

TREATMENT PRESCRIPTION

Primary Points: Liver (MA-SC5), Spleen (MA-IC), Stomach (MA-IC), and Heart (MA-IC).

Supplementary Points: Sān Jiāo (MA-IC4), Endocrine (MA-IC3), Subcortex (MA-AT1), Adrenal Gland (MA-T), Ear Shén Mén (MA-TF1), and Root of Ear Vagus (MA-PS).

THERAPEUTIC METHODS

Ear Acupuncture: Select two or three primary points together with one or two supplementary points. Use needle scratching with mild stimulation and retain needles for 30 minutes. Treat once per day. Begin treatment on a single ear and change to the opposite ear every other day. One treatment course is ten days; allow two or three days between treatment courses.

Ear Acupressure: Select the same points as above. Press the seeds three to five times, two to three minutes each time. Begin treatment on a single ear and change to the opposite ear every five to seven days.

Allergic Purpura

TREATMENT PRESCRIPTION

Primary Points: Spleen (MA-IC), Lung (MA-IC1), Heart (MA-IC), and Stomach (MA-IC).

Supplementary Points: Kidney (MA-SC), Subcortex (MA-AT1), Ear Shén Mén (MA-TF1), and Endocrine (MA-IC3).

THERAPEUTIC METHODS

Ear Acupuncture: Select two or three primary points together with one or two supplementary points. Retain the needles 30 to 60 minutes and manipulate every 10 to 15 minutes, using needle scratching and rotation. Treat once per day. Begin treatment on a single ear and change to the opposite ear every other day. One treatment course is ten days; allow two or three days between treatment courses.

Ear Acupressure: Select the same points as above. Press the seeds three to five times a day, two to three minutes each time. Begin treatment on a single ear and change to the opposite ear every five to seven days.

NOTES

- Try to discover the allergen during treatment.
- Ear acupuncture is also effective for treating recurrent allergic purpura.

EXTERNAL DISEASES

Lumbago

TREATMENT PRESCRIPTION 1

Primary Points: Ear Apex (MA-H6).

THERAPEUTIC METHOD

Medicine Injection: The patient should be seated. The ear apexes are sterilized, and 0.5 ml of Novocain is slowly injected into the prescribed point on both ears. Treat once per day.

NOTES

• This method is most effective in healing acute lumbar sprains.

TREATMENT PRESCRIPTION 2

Primary Points: Ear Shén Mén (MA-TF1), and Lumbosacral Vertebrae (MA-AH).

THERAPEUTIC METHOD

Ear Acupuncture: Needle Ear Shén Mén (MA-TF1) in the left ear first regardless of which side of the lumbus is most painful. Rotate the needle in one direction using strong stimulation for a few seconds, then needle Lumbosacral Vertebrae (MA-AH) in the same ear. Retain the needles for 30 minutes and manipulate every 10 minutes. After withdrawing the needles, have the patient gently bend at the waist or rotate his trunk for three to five minutes. If the patient continues to have pain, repeat the treatment in the right ear. The patient should rest in bed for two hours following treatment. Treat once per day until lumbago is healed.

NOTES

• This method is mainly used to treat acute lumbago.

TREATMENT PRESCRIPTION 3

Primary Points: Lumbosacral Vertebrae (MA-AH), Ear Shén Mén (MA-TF1), and Kidney (MA-SC).

Supplementary Points: Liver (MA-SC5), Sympathetic (MA-AH7), Subcortex (MA-AT1), and Adrenal Gland (MA-T).

THERAPEUTIC METHODS

Ear Acupuncture: Use all the primary points together with one or two supplementary points. Retain the needles 30 to 60 minutes and manipulate every 10 to 15 minutes, using needle scratching and rotation. Treat once per day. Begin treatment on a single ear and change to the opposite ear every other day. One treatment course is seven to ten days.

Ear Acupressure: Select the same points as above. Press the seeds three to five times a day, two to three minutes each time. Begin treatment on a single ear and change to the opposite ear every five to seven days.

NOTES

• Prescription 3 is mainly used to treat chronic lumbago.

Cervical Spondylopathy

TREATMENT PRESCRIPTION

Primary Points: Cervical Vertebrae (MA-AH8), Sympathetic (MA-AH7), and Ear Shén Mén (MA-TF1).

Supplementary Points: Occiput (MA-AT), Liver (MA-SC5), Kidney (MA-SC), Subcortex (MA-AT1), Adrenal Gland (MA-T), and corresponding points.

THERAPEUTIC METHODS

Ear Acupuncture: Use all the primary points together with one or two supplementary points. Retain the needles 30 minutes and manipulate every 10 minutes, using lifting and thrusting and needle rotation. Treat once per day. Begin treatment on a single ear and change to the opposite ear every other day. One treatment course is seven to ten days; allow two or three days between treatment courses.

Ear Acupressure: Select the same points as above. Affix vaccaria seeds and press them three to five times per day, two to three minutes each time. Begin treatment on a single ear and change to the opposite ear every five to seven days.

NOTES

- Cervical spondylopathy responds particularly well to treatment using ear acupuncture.
- Nodules or tenderness can be found on the affected cervical vertebrae.

Acute Sprain and Contusion

TREATMENT PRESCRIPTION

Primary Points: Ear Shén Mén (MA-TF1) and Subcortex (MA-AT1).

Supplementary Points: Liver (MA-SC5), Kidney (MA-SC), Spleen (MA-IC), Ear Apex (MA-H6), Endocrine (MA-IC3), and corresponding points.

THERAPEUTIC METHODS

Ear Acupuncture: Use all the primary points together with one or two supplementary points. For example, add Liver (MA-SC5) for injured tendons; add Spleen (MA-IC) if muscles are injured; add Ear Apex (MA-H6) and Endocrine (MA-IC3) for swelling and ecchymoma. Treat both ears simultaneously, using strong stimulation by applying lifting and thrusting and needle rotation. Retain the needles 30 to 60 minutes and manipulate every 10 to 15 minutes. The patient should move the affected area each time manipulation is done. Treat once per day until all symptoms are relieved.

Needle Implantation: Select the same points as above. Press the implanted needles three to five times a day, two to three minutes each time. Begin treatment on a single ear and change to the opposite ear every five to seven days.

Stiff Neck/Crick in the Neck

TREATMENT PRESCRIPTION

Primary Points: Neck (MA-AH10) and Ear Shén Mén (MA-TF1).

Supplementary Points: Cervical Vertebrae (MA-AH8), Subcortex (MA-AT1), and Adrenal Gland (MA-T).

THERAPEUTIC METHOD

Ear Acupuncture: Use all the primary points together with one or two supplementary points. Insert needles at sensitive spots at Neck (MA-AH10), Ear Shén Mén (MA-TF1), and Cervical Vertebrae (MA-AH8), using strong stimulation by applying needle scratching and rotation. Tell the patient to move the neck during manipulation until the manifestations are relieved, then retain the needles for 30 minutes, manipulating every 10 minutes. Treat once per day. In general, crick in the neck can be healed with two to five treatments.

CASE STUDY: CRICK IN THE NECK

Ding, a 40-year-old male, suffered from a stiff neck with limited range of motion since waking up the morning of his initial visit. The neck pain was on the right side and radiated to the right shoulder and upper back. Physical examination showed tightness on the trapezius muscle.

Treatment Prescription: Neck (MA-AH10), Occiput (MA-AT), Liver (MA-SC5), Kidney (MA-SC), Spleen (MA-IC), and Ear Shén Mén (MA-TF1).

Therapeutic Method: Needling all the above points on both ears with strong stimulation. The needles were retained for 30 minutes, and the patient was instructed to rotate his neck during needling.

Treatment Results: The neck pain started to go away after 10 minutes of treatment. The stiffness and limited range of motion were completely relieved after 30 minutes.

Comments: 1. Ear acupuncture is effective for relieving pain. The treatment of stiff and painful neck should include moving the neck while needling for better results.

2. The earlier the treatment is applied, the better the therapeutic result is. For crick in the neck three days after onset that is complicated with myofascitis, ear acupuncture itself cannot be expected to make a satisfactory treatment.

Frozen Shoulder

TREATMENT PRESCRIPTION

Primary Points: Shoulder (MA-SF4), Ear Shén Mén (MA-TF1), and Adrenal Gland (MA-T).

Supplementary Points: Clavicle (MA-SF5), Subcortex (MA-AT1), Spleen (MA-IC), Liver (MA-SC5), Kidney (MA-SC), and Endocrine (MA-IC3).

THERAPEUTIC METHODS

Ear Acupuncture: Use all the primary points together with one or two supplementary points. Retain the needles 30 to 60 minutes and manipulate every 10 to 15 minutes using needle scratching and rotation. Treat once per day. Begin treatment on a single ear and change to the opposite ear every other day. One treatment course is seven to ten days.

Electroacupuncture: Selection and insertion are the same as for needling. Connect the inserted needles to a stimulator for 30 minutes using the intermittent wave setting. Treat once per day. One treatment course is seven to ten days; allow two to three days between treatment courses.

Ear Acupressure: Select the same points as above. Affix vaccaria seeds and press them three to five times a day, two to three minutes each time. Begin treatment on a single ear and change to the opposite ear every five to seven days.

NOTES

* Tell the patient to actively move the shoulder during treatment, gradually increasing the amount and range of movement.

Tennis Elbow

TREATMENT PRESCRIPTION

Primary Points: Elbow (MA-SF3) and Ear Shén Mén (MA-TF1).

Supplementary Points: Adrenal Gland (MA-T), Wrist (MA-SF2), Spleen (MA-IC), and Subcortex (MA-AT1).

THERAPEUTIC METHODS

Ear Acupuncture: Use all the primary points together with one or two supplementary points. Retain the needles 30 to 60 minutes and manipulate every 10 to 15 minutes, using needle scratching and rotation. Treat once per day. Begin treatment on a single ear and change to the opposite ear every other day. One treatment course is seven to ten days.

Ear Acupressure: Select the same points as above. Press the vaccaria seeds three to five times a day, two to three minutes each time. Begin treatment on a single ear and change to the opposite ear every five to seven days.

Facial Paralysis

TREATMENT PRESCRIPTION 1

Primary Points: Eye (MA-L1), Cheek (MA-L), Forehead (MA-AT), and Mouth (MA-IC5).

Supplementary Points: Liver (MA-SC5), Spleen (MA-IC), Stomach (MA-IC), Adrenal Gland (MA-T), Subcortex (MA-AT1), and Ear Shén Mén (MA-TF1).

THERAPEUTIC METHODS

Ear Acupuncture: Use all the primary points together with one or two supplementary points. In the acute stage, treat both ears simultaneously, using strong stimulation by applying lifting and thrusting and needle rotation. Retain the needles 60 minutes and manipulate every 15 minutes. Treat once per day. One treatment course is seven days; allow two or three days between treatment courses. During the restoration stage, treat each ear on an alternate day. Retain the needles 30 minutes and manipulate every 10 minutes. Treat once per day. One treatment course is ten days; allow two or three days between treatment courses.

Ear Acupressure: Select the same points as above. Press the seeds three to five times per day, two to three minutes for each time. Begin treatment on a single ear and change to the opposite ear every five to seven days.

TREATMENT PRESCRIPTION 2

Primary Points: Posterior surface of the auricle and Helix 1-6 (MA-H 1-6).

THERAPEUTIC METHOD

Bloodletting: Rub the external ear to make it congested with blood, then pull the auricle taut with the index finger and thumb of one hand, while holding the surgical knife with the other hand. Stab the vein on the surface of the ear with the tip of the knife and draw 2 to 3 ml of blood, then stop the bleeding. Next, choose two or three points from the helix, drawing one or two drops from each with a three-edged needle.

NOTES

- In general, for mild cases, one treatment using two to four veins on the posterior surface of the auricle is sufficient to relieve this disorder.

CASE STUDY: FACIAL PARALYSIS

Zhou, a 50-year-old female, reported that she had wakened one morning with sudden onset of deviated eyes and mouth and drooling from the corner of her mouth. Physical examination showed that the wrinkles on the right side of the forehead had disappeared and inability to close the eyelid of the right side; the right nasolabial groove was gone and the mouth deviated to the left side. The diagnosis was "Bell's palsy."

Treatment Prescription: Cheek (MA-L), *Sān Jiāo* (MA-IC4), Liver (MA-SC5), Central Rim (MA-AT), Adrenal Gland (MA-T), and Subcortex (MA-AT1).

Therapeutic Method: Needling at all the above points, once per day, with 30 minutes of needle retention for each treatment. Both ears were treated simultaneously.

Treatment Results: After five treatments the right eyelid could close flexibly, the right nasolabial groove appeared, and drooling was remarkably reduced. The symptoms were completely gone after 20 treatments.

Comments: 1. Early treatment with ear acupuncture can prevent the later development of spasms in the facial muscles.

2. The earlier treatment is given, the better the therapeutic results.

3. One week or more after onset, ear acupuncture should be enhanced with body acupuncture for better effectiveness.

Facial Spasm

TREATMENT PRESCRIPTION

Primary Points: Eye (MA-L1), Cheek (MA-L), Ear Shén Mén (MA-TF1), and Mouth (MA-IC5).

Supplementary Points: Liver (MA-SC5), Subcortex (MA-AT1), Spleen (MA-IC), and Ear Apex (MA-H6).

THERAPEUTIC METHODS

Ear Acupuncture: Select two or three primary points together with one or two supplementary points. Retain the needles for 30 to 60 minutes and manipulate every 10 to 15 minutes, using needle scratching and rotation. Treat once per day. Begin treatment on a single ear and change to the opposite ear every other day. One treatment course is seven to ten days; allow two or three days between treatment courses.

Ear Acupressure: Select the same points as above. Press the seeds three to five times per day, two to three minutes each time. Begin treatment on a single ear and change to the opposite ear every five to seven days.

Intercostal Neuralgia

TREATMENT PRESCRIPTION

Primary Points: Chest (MA-AH11), Liver (MA-SC5), and Ear Shén Mén (MA-TF1).

Supplementary Points: Subcortex (MA-AT1), Occiput (MA-AT), and Adrenal Gland (MA-T).

THERAPEUTIC METHODS

Electroacupuncture: Detect the most sensitive spot around Chest (MA-AH11), and then needle it with a filiform needle. In most cases, intercostal neuralgia pain should be relieved only a few seconds after needle insertion; if not, withdraw the needle and insert needles at Liver (MA-SC5), Ear Shén Mén (MA-TF1), and Subcortex (MA-AT1); connect the needles to an electroacupuncture apparatus for 30 minutes using the intermittent wave setting. Begin treatment on a single ear and change to the opposite ear every other day. One treatment course is seven days; allow two or three days between treatment courses.

Ear Acupressure: Use all the primary points together with one or two supplementary points. Affix vaccaria seeds and press them three to five times per day, two to three minutes each time, or until pain is relieved. Begin treatment on a single ear and change to the opposite ear every five to seven days. Force should gradually be increased while pressing, and the patient should intentionally breathe deeply or cough during the treatment.

Sciatica

TREATMENT PRESCRIPTION 1

Primary Points: Sciatic Nerve (MA-AH6) and Lumbosacral Vertebrae (MA-AH).

THERAPEUTIC METHOD

Ear Acupuncture: Use both points, applying strong stimulation by applying lifting and thrusting and needle rotation. Retain the needles for one to two hours. Treat once per day. Begin treatment on a single ear and change to the opposite ear every other day. One treatment course is seven days; allow two or three days between treatment courses.

TREATMENT PRESCRIPTION 2

Primary Points: Sciatic Nerve (MA-AH6), Lumbosacral Vertebrae (MA-AH), and Ear Shén Mén (MA-TF1).

Supplementary Points: Hip (MA-AH4), Knee (MA-AH3), Adrenal Gland (MA-T), Subcortex (MA-AT1), and Kidney (MA-SC).

THERAPEUTIC METHOD

Ear Acupressure: Use all the primary points together with one or two supplementary points. Press the vaccaria seeds three to five times a day, two to three minutes each time. Begin treatment on a single ear and change to the opposite ear every five to seven days.

Head Injury Sequelae

TREATMENT PRESCRIPTION

Primary Points: Kidney (MA-SC), Subcortex (MA-AT1), Occiput (MA-AT), and Forehead (MA-AT).

Supplementary Points: Cervical Vertebrae (MA-AH8), Heart (MA-IC), Liver (MA-SC5), Sympathetic (MA-AH7), and Ear Shén Mén (MA-TF1).

THERAPEUTIC METHODS

Needle Implantation: Select two or three primary points together with one or two supplementary points. After sterilization, implant intradermal needles at the selected points. Press the implanted needles three to five times per day, two to three minutes each time. Begin treatment on a single ear and change to the opposite ear every five to seven days.

Ear Acupressure: Select three to five primary points and add supplementary points as needed. Press the vaccaria seeds three to five times per day, two to three minutes each time. Begin treatment on a single ear and change to the opposite ear every five to seven days.

NOTES

• The sooner ear acupuncture is started after post-head injury syndrome is diagnosed, the better the therapeutic effect.

• Even after all symptoms are relieved, one or two additional courses of treatment should be given.

Phantom Limb Pain

TREATMENT PRESCRIPTION

Primary Points: Ear Shén Mén (MA-TF1), Subcortex (MA-AT1), Adrenal Gland (MA-T), Forehead (MA-AT), and corresponding points.

THERAPEUTIC METHODS

Needle Implantation: Select two or three prescribed points. Embed the intradermal needles into the points until soreness, numbness, distention, or heaviness is felt. Press the implanted needles three to five times per day, three to five minutes each time, or until pain is relieved. Begin treatment on a single ear and change to the opposite ear every three to five days in winter, or every five to seven days in summer; or treat both ears simultaneously every two or three days.

NOTE

- According to TCM, the channels converge in the ears. Therefore, irregular circulation of qì and blood after amputation will be reflected in the ears.

Cholelithiasis

TREATMENT PRESCRIPTION

Primary Points: Liver (MA-SC5), Pancreas/Gallbladder (MA-SC6), and Duodenum (MA-SC1).

Supplementary Points: Add Ear Apex (MA-H6) for fever; add Esophagus (MA-IC6) and Stomach (MA-IC) for nausea and vomiting; add Sympathetic (MA-AH7), and Ear Shén Mén (MA-TF1) for severe pain; add *Sān Jiāo* (MA-IC4) and Large Intestine (MA-SC4) for constipation and distention of abdomen.

THERAPEUTIC METHODS

Ear Acupuncture: Use all the primary points together with one or two supplementary points, according to the patient's condition. Retain the needles 30 minutes and manipulate every 10 minutes, using strong stimulation by applying lifting and thrusting and needle rotation. Treat once per day. Begin treatment on a single ear and change to the opposite ear every other day. One treatment course is seven to ten days; allow two or three days between treatment courses. For those with severe pain, treatment twice per day is recommended.

Ear Acupressure: Select the same points as above. Use vaccaria seeds or magnetic beads. Press the seeds or beads three to five times per day, two to three minutes each time. Begin treatment on a single ear and change to the opposite ear every five to seven days.

NOTES

- Bloodletting with a three-edged needle is done in the ear apex if the patient has a fever.

- The factors that determine therapeutic effectiveness of ear acupuncture on cholelithiasis include:

Sensation — A better therapeutic effect results if the patient has a strong reaction to ear acupuncture.

Constitution — Those with a strong constitution or those who engage in manual labor experience a better therapeutic effect from ear acupuncture, as physical exertion helps the movement of the gallbladder.

Gallbladder function — Treatment of cholelithiasis by ear acupuncture is more effective if the gallbladder has no other abnormalities of shape or function.

Size, shape and adhesiveness of gallstones — In general, gallstones that are smaller (i.e., with a diameter that is less than 10 mm), have smoother surfaces, and don't adhere to the gallbladder wall are more easily treated.

Location of gallstones — Gallstones that are in the common bile duct are easier to evacuate. Cystic stones or stones found in bile ducts in the liver are more difficult to evacuate.

Emotional condition of the patient — TCM considers emotional depression to have an especially strong effect on the liver and gallbladder. Therefore, ear acupuncture is far less effective in those with melancholy or psychological stress.

Stage of cholelithiasis — A better therapeutic effect is more frequently seen when cholelithiasis is treated in the acute stage rather than while it is in remission.

Weather — A better therapeutic effect is generally achieved in warmer rather than colder weather.

Chronic Appendicitis/Intestinal Welling

TREATMENT PRESCRIPTION

Primary Points: Appendix (MA-SC3), Large Intestine (MA-SC4), and Small Intestine (MA-SC2).

Supplementary Points: Add Rectum (MA-H2) and Lung (MA-IC1) for constipation; add Spleen (MA-IC) and Stomach (MA-IC) for abdominal distention and nausea; add Subcortex (MA-AT1) and Sympathetic (MA-AH7) for severe pain.

THERAPEUTIC METHODS

Ear Acupuncture: Use all the primary points together with supplementary points, according to the patient's condition. Retain the needles 30 to 60 minutes and manipulate every 10 to 15 minutes, using lifting and thrusting and needle rotation. Treat once per day. Begin treatment on a single ear and change to the opposite ear every other day. One treatment course is seven to ten days; allow two or three days between treatment courses. In severe cases, treatment can be given every four hours.

Ear Acupressure: Select the same points as above. Use vaccaria seeds in both ears at the beginning. Press the seeds three to five times a day, two to three minutes each time, until all symptoms are relieved; then treat only one ear, changing to the opposite ear every five to seven days.

Bloodletting: Prick with a three-edged needle or filiform needle at Ear Apex (MA-H6) or Helix 1-6 (MA-H 1-6) in both ears. This therapy is used for those suffering from an acute attack accompanied by fever.

Hemorrhoids

TREATMENT PRESCRIPTION

Primary Points: Anus (MA-H5), Large Intestine (MA-SC4), Small Intestine (MA-SC2), and Ear Shén Mén (MA-TF1).

Supplementary Points: Add Subcortex (MA-AT1) and sensitive spots for severe pain; add Pelvis (MA-TF) and Kidney (MA-SC) for lumbago or discomfort in lumbar area; add Sympathetic (MA-AH7) for excessive bleeding.

THERAPEUTIC METHODS

Ear Acupressure: Use all the primary points together with supplementary points, according to the patient's condition. Press the vaccaria seeds three to five times per day, two or three minutes each time. Begin treatment on a single ear and change to the opposite ear every five to seven days.

Prolapse of the Rectum

TREATMENT PRESCRIPTION

Primary Points: Anus (MA-H5), Large Intestine (MA-SC4), Spleen (MA-IC), and Subcortex (MA-AT1).

Supplementary Points: Add Lumbosacral (MA-AH) for soreness and pain in the lumbosacral area.

THERAPEUTIC METHODS

Ear Acupuncture: Needle Anus (MA-H5) connecting to Large Intestine (MA-SC4) using strong stimulation by applying lifting and thrusting and needle rotation; more moderate manipulations should be done at other points. Retain the needles 30 to 60 minutes and manipulate every 10 to 15 minutes. Treat once per day. Begin treatment on a single ear and change to the opposite ear every other day. One treatment course is seven to ten days; allow two or three days between treatment courses.

Electroacupuncture: Use the same points as above, but connect the needles to an electroacupuncture apparatus for 30 minutes. Choose continuous wave setting at a frequency of 200 Hz. Treat once per day. One treatment course is five to seven days.

Ear Acupressure: Select two or three points for each treatment. Press the vaccaria seeds three to five times per day, two to three minutes each time. Treat both ears simultaneously. One treatment course is five to seven days; allow two or three days between treatment courses.

Needle Implantation: Select two or three points for each treatment. Press the implanted needles three to five times per day, two to three minutes each time. Begin treatment on a single ear and change to the opposite ear every five to seven days. One treatment course is five to seven days; allow seven days between treatment courses.

NOTES

* Medicinal and surgical therapies should also be employed whenever prolapse of rectum results in prolapsed hemorrhoids, edema, or necrosis.

Acute Mastitis

TREATMENT PRESCRIPTION

Primary Points: Mammary Gland (MA-AH)[15], Chest (MA-AH11), and Endocrine (MA-IC3).

Supplementary Points: Add Ear Apex (MA-H6) for fever; add Liver (MA-SC5) and Adrenal Gland (MA-T) for severe distention of the affected breast and disturbance of milk; add Spleen (MA-IC) and Stomach (MA-IC) for poor appetite and weak constitution.

THERAPEUTIC METHODS

Ear Acupuncture: Use all the primary points together with one or two supplementary points, according to the patient's condition. Treat both ears simultaneously, applying strong stimulation by lifting and thrusting and needle rotation. Retain the needles 30 to 60 minutes and manipulate every 10 to 15 minutes. Treat one or two times per day.

Needle Implantation: Select the same points as above. After routine sterilization, implant intradermal needles at the selected points. Press the needles three to five times per day, two to three minutes each time. Begin treatment on a single ear and change to the opposite ear every five to seven days.

---

[15] Mammary Gland (MA-AH) is located by palpating for a sensitive point on Chest (MA-AH11).

Bloodletting: Use bloodletting for cases with fever and severe breast pain. Prick to bleed at Ear Apex (MA-H6) and Mammary Gland (MA-AH).

NOTES

- All the above therapies are recommended for the early stage of acute mastitis.
- Patients with generalized infection and local pyogenic formation should be treated with anti-inflammatory medicines that drain pus.

Urinary Stone

TREATMENT PRESCRIPTION

Primary Points: Kidney (MA-SC) and Ureter (MA-SC7).

Supplementary Points: Add Ear Shén Mén (MA-TF1) and Subcortex (MA-AT1) for renal colic; add Sympathetic (MA-AH7) and Adrenal Gland (MA-T) for urine retaining blood; add Urethra (MA-H3) and Lung (MA-IC1) for disturbance or retention of urine; add Spleen (MA-IC) and Stomach (MA-IC) for poor appetite and listlessness.

THERAPEUTIC METHODS

Ear Acupressure: Select all primary points together with one or two supplementary points. Press the vaccaria seeds three to five times per day; continue pressing until the ear feels hot. Exercise and drink 300 to 500 ml of water before treatment to aid in the evacuation of the calculus. Begin treatment on a single ear and change to the opposite ear every five to seven days.

Electroacupuncture: Use all the primary points together with supplementary points, according to the patient's condition. Insert filiform needles into points, using strong stimulation. Connect the needles to an electroacupuncture apparatus for 30 to 60 minutes using a frequency of 200hz at the intermittent wave setting. Treat twice per day for those with severe pain, once per day for common cases. Begin treatment on a single ear and change to the opposite ear every other day.

GYNECOLOGICAL AND OBSTETRIC DISORDERS

Dysmenorrhea/Menstrual Pain

TREATMENT PRESCRIPTION

Primary Points: Pelvis (MA-TF), Endocrine (MA-IC3), and Ear Shén Mén (MA-TF1).

Supplementary Points: Internal Reproductive Organs (MA-TF), Liver (MA-SC5), Sympathetic (MA-AH7), Root of Ear Vagus (MA-PS), Subcortex (MA-AT1), and Stomach (MA-IC).

THERAPEUTIC METHODS

Ear Acupuncture: Use all the primary points together with one or two supplementary points, according to the patient's condition. For example, add Sympathetic (MA-AH7) and Subcortex (MA-AT1) for severe abdominal pain; add Stomach (MA-IC) for nausea and vomiting. Treat both ears simultaneously, using strong stimulation by applying lifting and thrusting and needle rotation. Continue manipulating until pain is relieved, then retain the needles an additional 30 to 60 minutes, manipulating every 10 to 15 minutes. Treat once or twice a day until all symptoms are relieved.

Ear Acupressure: Select the same points as above. Affix vaccaria seeds and press them three to five times per day; continue pressing until pain is completely relieved.

CASE STUDY: DYSMENORRHEA

Qian, an 18-year-old female, had suffered from severe lower abdominal pain for the last several years, with lumbosacral soreness at the beginning of each period. The pain was automatically relieved on the second day of each period. She had heavy menstrual flow with blood clots. The diagnosis was "primary dysmenorrhea."

Treatment Prescription: Internal Reproductive Organs (MA-TF), Liver (MA-SC5), Kidney (MA-SC), Endocrine (MA-IC3), Subcortex (MA-AT1), and Ear Shén Mén (MA-TF1).

Therapeutic Method: All the above points were needled with strong stimulation on both ears simultaneously.

Treatment Results: Abdominal pain was greatly relieved 10 minutes after needling. Pain was completely gone after 30 minutes of treatment.

Comments: 1. Treatment of dysmenorrhea with ear acupuncture can only relieve pain as it occurs. For better results, the treatment should be done three days before the period with seed acupressure at all the above points on both ears simultaneously. The patient should be told to press the seeds three to five times per day during the treatment.

　　　2. Psychological therapy for relieving nervousness and PMS symptoms can increase the therapeutic effect of ear acupuncture.

CASE STUDY: PREMENSTRUAL SYNDROME (PMS)

Chou, an 18-year-old female, reported that each month over the last two years she would have irritability, impatience, emotional depression, distention and pain in both breasts, and slightly puffy face. These symptom would always appear three to five days before her period and disappear right after the onset of menses. A physical examination revealed no explanation for this problem. The diagnosis was "premenstrual syndrome."

Treatment Prescription: Internal Reproductive Organs (MA-TF), Liver (MA-SC5), Kidney (MA-SC), Adrenal Gland (MA-T), Endocrine (MA-IC3), Ear Shén Mén (MA-TF1), and Subcortex (MA-AT1).

Therapeutic Method: Seed acupressure was applied to all the above points from seven days before the period until the period was complete. Both ears were treated simultaneously, twice a week. The patient was told to press the seeds three to five times per day during the treatment.

Treatment Results: All the symptoms were reduced by treatments during the first two cycles; they were completely relieved after treatment through six cycles. To maintain the therapeutic result, further treatment was given for three more cycles. According to follow-up examinations, the PMS did not recur for more than one year after the treatment.

Amenorrhea

TREATMENT PRESCRIPTION

Primary Points: Internal Reproductive Organs (MA-TF), Endocrine (MA-IC3), Subcortex (MA-AT1), and Central Rim (MA-AT).

Supplementary Points: Sympathetic (MA-AH7), Liver (MA-SC5), Kidney (MA-SC), Heart (MA-IC), Spleen (MA-IC), Stomach (MA-IC), and Ear Shén Mén (MA-TF1).

THERAPEUTIC METHODS

Ear Acupuncture: Select two or three primary points together with one or two supplementary points. Retain the needles 30 to 60 minutes and manipulate every 10 to 15 minutes, using needle scratching and rotation. Treat once per day. Begin treatment on a single ear and change to the opposite ear every other day. One treatment course is seven days; allow two or three days between treatment courses.

Ear Acupressure: Select the same points as above. Press the vaccaria seeds three to five times per day, three to five minutes each time. Begin treatment on a single ear and change to the opposite ear every five to seven days.

Notes

- Ear acupuncture is effective by itself in treating functional amenor-rhea, but organic amenorrhea should be treated in combination with other therapies.

> **Case Study: Amenorrhea**
>
> Xu, a 17-year-old female, reported that she had been experiencing amenorrhea for the last six months. There were no other symptoms or signs. The diagnosis was "amenorrhea due to ovarian dysfunction."
>
> **Treatment Prescription:** Internal Reproductive Organs (MA-TF), Liver (MA-SC5), Kidney (MA-SC), Spleen (MA-IC), Subcortex (MA-AT1), and Endocrine (MA-IC3).
>
> **Therapeutic Method:** Seed acupressure was applied to all the above points. The ears were treated alternately, switching ears twice a week. The patient was told to press the seeds three to five times per day during the treatment.
>
> **Treatment Results:** The patient's period started after the eighth treatment. Afterwards, two treatments of seed acupressure were given in the five days before the period. The patient was told to press the seeds three to five times per day during the treatment. Her menses returned to normal after three months.
>
> **Comment:** Ear acupuncture is quite effective for dysfunctional ovarian amenorrhea.

Irregular Menstruation/Menstrual Irregularities

Treatment Prescription

Primary Points: Internal Reproductive Organs (MA-TF), Endocrine (MA-IC3), Liver (MA-SC5), and Kidney (MA-SC).

Supplementary Points: Spleen (MA-IC), Sympathetic (MA-AH7), Subcortex (MA-AT1), Ear Shén Mén (MA-TF1), and Central Rim (MA-AT).

Therapeutic Methods

Ear Acupuncture: Select two or three primary points together with one or two supplementary points. Retain the needles 30 to 60 minutes and manipulate every 10 to 15 minutes, using needle scratching and rotation. Treat once per day. Begin treatment on a single ear and change to the opposite ear every other day. One treatment course is seven to ten days; allow two to three days between treatment courses.

Ear Acupressure: Select the same points as above. Press the vaccaria seeds three to five times per day, two to three minutes each time. Begin treatment on a single ear and change to the opposite ear every five to seven days.

NOTES

- Ear acupuncture should be given every month and applied regularly during the five to seven days preceding menstruation and the five to seven days following menstruation.
- Ear acupuncture is more effective for treating functional irregular menstruation because it is bi-directional, and so regulates endocrine function.

CASE STUDY: IRREGULAR MENSTRUATION

Dong, a 20-year-old female, reported that for six months she had prolonged menstrual cycles, heavy menses that was dark red in color, and a dull pain in the lower abdomen. The diagnosis was "Irregular Menstruation (Prolonged Cycle)."

Treatment Prescription: Internal Reproductive Organs (MA-TF), Liver (MA-SC5), Kidney (MA-SC), Spleen (MA-IC), Subcortex (MA-AT1), and Endocrine (MA-IC3).

Therapeutic Method: Seed acupressure was applied to all the above points. The ears were treated alternately, switching ears twice a week. The patient was told to press the seeds three to five times per day during the treatment.

Treatment Results: Menses turned normal after three months. To enhance the therapeutic results, the patient continued treatment for a total of six months.

Comment: Ear acupuncture is effective in regulating ovarian function, but for the treatment of irregular menstruation, a longer treatment course is needed.

Leukorrhea/Vaginal Discharge

TREATMENT PRESCRIPTION

Primary Points: Internal Reproductive Organs (MA-TF), Kidney (MA-SC), and Spleen (MA-IC).

Supplementary Points: Add Wind Stream (MA-SF) for itching in the vulva and vagina; add Subcortex (MA-AT1) for pain in the lower abdomen; add Endocrine (MA-IC3) for profuse, thin, and clear vaginal discharge; add Liver (MA-SC5) and *Sān Jiāo* (MA-IC4) for foul-smelling leukorrhea with thick pus, or for short voidings of reddish urine; add Ear Apex (MA-H6) and Adrenal Gland (MA-T) for fever.

THERAPEUTIC METHODS

Needle Implantation: Select two or three primary points together with one or two supplementary points. Implant needles at the selected points. Press the needles three to five times per day, two to three minutes each time. Begin treatment on a single ear and change to the opposite ear every five to seven days.

Ear Acupressure: Select all primary points together with supplementary points, according to the patient's condition. Press the vaccaria seeds three to five times per day, two to three minutes each time. Begin treatment on a single ear and change to the opposite ear every five to seven days.

CASE STUDY: LEUKORRHEA

Sun, a 30-year-old female, reported that for the past year she had endured profuse vaginal discharge following an abortion. The discharge was sticky, yellowish, and odorless; there was also soreness and pain of the lumbar region as well as listlessness. Physical and gynecological examinations revealed no explanations for this problem. The diagnosis was "pelvic inflammation."

Treatment Prescription: Internal Reproductive Organs (MA-TF), Pelvis (MA-TF), Adrenal Gland (MA-T), Endocrine (MA-IC3), Sympathetic (MA-AH7), and Ear Shén Mén (MA-TF1).

Therapeutic Method: Seed acupressure was applied to all the above points. The ears were treated alternately, switching ears twice a week. The patient was told to press the seeds three to five times per day during the treatment.

Treatment Results: The amount of vaginal discharge was remarkably reduced and all the other symptoms were relieved after treatment for 15 days. All the symptoms were completely gone after one month.

Comment: Ear acupuncture has the best therapeutic results for leukorrhea due to spleen vacuity or spleen-kidney vacuity.

Surgical Abortion Syndrome

TREATMENT PRESCRIPTION

Primary Points: Internal Reproductive Organs (MA-TF), Sympathetic (MA-AH7), and Endocrine (MA-IC3).

Supplementary Points: Add Adrenal Gland (MA-T) and Central Rim (MA-AT) for low blood pressure; add Ear Center (MA-H1) for excessive bleeding; add Ear Shén Mén (MA-TF1) and Occiput (MA-AT) for severe pain.

THERAPEUTIC METHODS

Medicine Injection: Five minutes prior to the operation, inject 1 ml of 2% lidocaine into Internal Reproductive Organs (MA-TF) in the right ear. This therapy can promote contraction of the uterus and relaxation of the ostium of the uterus, relieve pain, and reduce bleeding.

Ear Acupuncture: Select two or three primary points together with one or two supplementary points. Retain the needles 30 to 60 minutes and manipulate every 10 to 15 minutes, using needle scratching and rotation. Treat once per day. Begin treatment on a single ear and change to the opposite ear every other day. One treatment course is seven days; allow two or three days between treatment courses.

CASE STUDY: SURGICAL ABORTION SYNDROME

Li, a 30-year-old female, had surgical abortion for a 40-day pregnancy. During the dilation and curettage with suction procedure she had nausea, vomiting, sudden paleness of face, cold sweats, and a thready, feeble pulse. Her heart beat was 60/min. The clinical diagnosis was "surgical abortion syndrome."

Treatment Prescription: Mouth (MA-IC5), Liver (MA-SC5), Heart (MA-IC), Adrenal Gland (MA-T), and Endocrine (MA-IC3).

Therapeutic Method: All the above points were needled with strong stimulation; both ears were treated.

Treatment Results: Nausea and vomiting stopped after 3 minutes, and all other symptoms started improving. The patient's heart beat returned to 70/min.

Comment: As an empirical point, Mouth (MA-IC5) is important in the treatment of this case because it is located where the auricular branch of the vagus nerve travels through the ear. All the symptoms in this case were caused by vagus nerve reflex due to pulling and stretching of internal organs during surgery.

Postpartum Urine Retention

TREATMENT PRESCRIPTION

Primary Points: Bladder (MA-SC8), Kidney (MA-SC), *Sān Jiāo* (MA-IC4), and Central Rim (MA-AT).

Supplementary Points: Add Spleen (MA-IC) for poor appetite, listlessness, and pale face; add Liver (MA-SC5) and Sympathetic (MA-AH7) for pain and distention in the lower abdomen and restlessness; add Lung (MA-IC1) for shortness of breath and lack of desire to speak.

THERAPEUTIC METHODS

Medicine Injection: Inject 0.2 ml of vitamin B_{12} into each of Kidney (MA-SC), Bladder (MA-SC8), and Central Rim (MA-AT). Begin treatment on a single ear and change to the opposite ear every other day.

Ear Acupuncture: Select two or three primary points together with one or two supplementary points. Retain the needles 30 to 60 minutes and manipulate every 10 to 15 minutes, using needle scratching and rotation. Treat once per day. Begin treatment on a single ear and change to the opposite ear every other day. One treatment course is seven days; allow two or three days between treatment courses.

CASE STUDY: POSTPARTUM URINE RETENTION

Sheng, a 27-year-old female, reported that she had failed to urinate for six hours after birth of her baby; she had severe distention in the lower abdomen. Physical examination showed distention of the urinary bladder and dullness upon tapping. The clinical diagnosis was "postpartum urine retention."

Treatment Prescription: Bladder (MA-SC8), Kidney (MA-SC), Spleen (MA-IC), Lung (MA-IC1), *Sān Jiāo* (MA-IC4), and Subcortex (MA-AT1).

Therapeutic Method: Needle all the above points in both ears with strong stimulation.

Treatment Results: The patient urinated once after 10 minutes. Her urination returned to normal thereafter.

Comments: 1. With urine retention, the patient normally manifests anxiety and irritability. But the points for calming, such as Ear Shén Mén (MA-TF1) and Occiput (MA-AT), should not be used because they may cause storage of urine.

2. Ear acupuncture is significantly helpful for healing postpartum urine retention. In general, it is effective for paralytic urine retention, but not for the obstructed type.

Postpartum Hypolactation

TREATMENT PRESCRIPTION

Primary Points: Mammary Gland (MA-AH), Endocrine (MA-IC3), and Central Rim (MA-AT).

Supplementary Points: Add Spleen (MA-IC) and Stomach (MA-IC) for qì and blood vacuity; add Liver (MA-SC5) and Sympathetic (MA-AH7) for stagnation of liver qì.

THERAPEUTIC METHODS

Ear Acupuncture: Select two or three primary points together with supplementary points, according to the patient's condition. Retain the needles 30 to 60 minutes and manipulate every 10 to 15 minutes, using needle scratching and rotation. Treat once per day. Begin treatment on a single ear and change to the opposite ear every other day. One treatment course is seven days; allow two or three days between treatment courses.

Ear Acupressure: Use all the primary points together with supplementary points, according to the patient's condition. Press the vaccaria seeds three to five times per day, three to five minutes each time. Begin treatment on a single ear and change to the opposite ear every five to seven days.

Prolapse of the Uterus/Yīn Protrusion

TREATMENT PRESCRIPTION

Primary Points: Internal Reproductive Organs (MA-TF), Subcortex (MA-AT1), Spleen (MA-IC), and Kidney (MA-SC).

Supplementary Points: Sympathetic (MA-AH7), External Genitals (MA-H4), and Ear Apex (MA-H6).

THERAPEUTIC METHODS

Electroacupuncture: Select two or three primary points together with one or two supplementary points. Insert filiform needles into the auricular perichondrium, using needle scratching and rotation of the needles for two minutes, then connect the needles to an electroacupuncture apparatus using a continuous wave setting at a frequency of 180hz. Continue stimulation for 30 minutes. Set current intensity to patient tolerance. Treat once per day. Begin treatment on a single ear and change to the opposite ear every other day. One treatment course is ten days.

Needle Implantation: Select two or three primary points together with one or two supplementary points. Implant needles at the selected points. Press the implanted needles three to five times per day, two to three minutes each time. Begin treatment on a single ear and change to the opposite ear every five to seven days.

Bloodletting: Prick Ear Apex (MA-H6) with a three-edged needle and draw three drops of blood. Treat once per day for three successive days. This method is effective for those with an infection.

Climacteric Syndrome (Menopause)

TREATMENT PRESCRIPTION

Primary Points: Internal Reproductive Organs (MA-TF), Subcortex (MA-AT1), Kidney (MA-SC), and Endocrine (MA-IC3).

Supplementary Points: Add Heart (MA-IC) and Ear Shén Mén (MA-TF1) for palpitations and insomnia; add Liver (MA-SC5) and Sympathetic (MA-AH7) for irritability and shortness of temper; add Occiput (MA-AT) for dizziness and tinnitus.

THERAPEUTIC METHODS

Ear Acupressure: Select three or four primary points together with supplementary points, according to the patient's condition. Press the vaccaria seeds three to five times per day, three to five minutes each time. Begin treatment on a single ear and change to the opposite ear every five to seven days.

Ear Acupuncture: Select two or three primary points together with one or two supplementary points. Retain the needles 30 to 60 minutes and manipulate every 10 to 15 minutes, using needle scratching and rotation. Treat once per day. Begin treatment on a single ear and change to the opposite ear every other day. One treatment course is seven to ten days; allow two or three days between treatment courses.

CASE STUDY: MENOPAUSAL SYNDROME

Zhao, a 52-year-old female, had suffered for the last three years from irregular menses with heavy flow, dizziness, insomnia, spontaneous sweating, irritability, and paroxysmal facial flushing. The diagnosis was "menopausal syndrome." There had been no relief from hormone treatment that had lasted more than one year.

Treatment Prescription: Internal Reproductive Organs (MA-TF), Kidney (MA-SC), Liver (MA-SC5), Subcortex (MA-AT1), Endocrine (MA-IC3), Central Rim (MA-AT), and Anterior Ear Lobe (MA-L).

Therapeutic Method: Seed acupressure was applied to all the above points. The ears were treated alternately, switching ears every three days. The patient was told to press the seeds three to five times per day during the treatment.

Treatment Results: With four treatments the patient's insomnia improved and all other symptoms were better. With eight treatments the symptoms were all relieved and her emotions were stabilized. Another four treatments were applied to enhance the therapeutic results.

> **Comments:** 1. Menopausal syndrome patients usually have many symptoms to complain about. The selection of points should be based on the chief complaint.
>
> 2. Ear acupuncture can regulate the functions of vegetative nerves, but the treatment course can be one month or more.

PEDIATRIC DISORDERS

Infantile Bronchitis/Pediatric Coughing or Panting

TREATMENT PRESCRIPTION

Primary Points: Bronchii/Trachea (MA-IC2), Lung (MA-IC1), and Adrenal Gland (MA-T).

Supplementary Points: Add Apex of Antitragus (MA-AT)[16] for severe asthma; add Spleen (MA-IC) for profuse phlegm; add Ear Apex (MA-H6) for fever; add Sympathetic (MA-AH7) and Ear Shén Mén (MA-TF1) for irritability and persistent crying; add Kidney (MA-SC) for chronic cases.

THERAPEUTIC METHODS

Ear Acupuncture: Select two or three primary points together with one or two supplementary points. Retain the needles 30 to 60 minutes and manipulate every 10 to 15 minutes, using needle scratching and rotation. Treat once per day. Begin treatment on a single ear and change to the opposite ear every other day. One treatment course is seven to ten days; allow two or three days between treatment courses.

Bloodletting: Ear Apex (MA-H6) is treated on both ears simultaneously. Prick the points with a three-edged needle to draw two or three drops of blood. This is especially effective in those with high fever. Give one treatment a day until fever is reduced.

Ear Acupressure: Use all the primary points together with supplementary points, according to the patient's condition. Press the vaccaria

---

[16] We clinically denote this point as *Píng Chuǎn*. According to the WHO international standards schema, Apex of Antitragus (MA-AT) includes *Píng Chuǎn* (Calm Panting) and *Sāi Xiàn* (Parotid). In actual clinical practice it also includes *Gāo Wán* (Testicle). Apex of Antitragus is used as an area, not a specific point. Parotid is located on the inner aspect of Apex of Antitragus. Testicle is located on the anterior aspect, diagonally and posteriorly on a line from Parotid and just off Apex of Antitragus. Calm Panting is located further anteriorly along the same line, the same distance from Testicle as Testicle is from Parotid. If a patient has asthma, we palpate in this area; the tender spot is used as *Píng Chuǎn*. If a patient has parotitis, the tender spot in this area would be *Sāi Xiàn* (Parotid). The same thing will happen with *Gāo Wán* (Testicle). Some texts do not list *Píng Chuǎn*, *Gāo Wán*, and *Sāi Xiàn* and instead list *Duì Píng Jiān* (Apex of Antitragus) as a point.

seeds three to five times per day, three to five minutes each time. Begin treatment on a single ear and change to the opposite ear every five to seven days.

Pediatric Fever

TREATMENT PRESCRIPTION

Primary Points: Ear Apex (MA-H6) and Adrenal Gland (MA-T).

Supplementary Points: Add Occiput (MA-AT), Forehead (MA-AT), and Temple (MA-AT) for headache; add Liver (MA-SC5) and Ear Shén Mén (MA-TF1) for prodromal signs of convulsion; add Lung (MA-IC1) and Bronchii/Trachea (MA-IC2) for cough; add Pharynx and Larynx (MA-T3) and Tonsil (MA-L) for sore throat.

THERAPEUTIC METHODS

Bloodletting: For mild fevers, begin treatment at Ear Apex (MA-H6) on a single ear, then treat Adrenal Gland (MA-T), alternating ears every other day. Prick the point with a three-edged needle to draw three to five drops of blood. For high fevers, treat both ears simultaneously. Treat once per day until fever is reduced.

Ear Acupressure: Select all primary points together with supplementary points, according to the patient's condition. Press the vaccaria seeds three to five times per day, three to five minutes each time. Begin treatment on a single ear and change to the opposite ear every five to seven days.

NOTES

- In general, body temperature will be reduced 0.8-1.2° C one-half hour after bloodletting. It will return to normal after three treatments.
- Medicinal therapy may be needed if treatment by bloodletting is not effective.

(Pediatric) Aversion to Food

TREATMENT PRESCRIPTION

Primary Points: Stomach (MA-IC), Spleen (MA-IC), and Small Intestine (MA-SC2).

Supplementary Points: Add Large Intestine (MA-SC4) for abnormal stools; add Kidney (MA-SC) for dry and sparse hair; add Liver (MA-SC5) and Pancreas/Gallbladder (MA-SC6) for distention or discomfort in the abdomen.

THERAPEUTIC METHODS

Ear Acupressure: Use all the primary points together with one or two supplementary points, according to the patient's condition. Press the seeds three to five times per day, two to three minutes each time. Begin treatment on a single ear and change to the opposite ear every five to seven days.

Needle Implantation: Use all the primary points together with one or two supplementary points. Quickly implant intradermal needles at the selected points. Press the needles three to five times per day, two to three minutes each time. Begin treatment on a single ear and change to the opposite ear every five to seven days.

Infantile Diarrhea

TREATMENT PRESCRIPTION

Primary Points: Spleen (MA-IC), Stomach (MA-IC), Large Intestine (MA-SC4), and Small Intestine (MA-SC2).

Supplementary Points: Add *Sān Jiāo* (MA-IC4) and Endocrine (MA-IC3) for watery stools; add Sympathetic (MA-AH7) and Liver (MA-SC5) for vomiting and abdominal distention; add Subcortex (MA-AT1) and Adrenal Gland (MA-T) for mild fever and listlessness.

THERAPEUTIC METHODS

Ear Acupressure: Use all the primary points together with one or two supplementary points, according to the patient's condition. Press the seeds three to five times per day, two to three minutes each time. Begin treatment on a single ear and change to the opposite ear every five to seven days.

NOTES

- Ear acupuncture is recommended for the milder type of diarrhea. Medicinal therapy should be given for the more severe types of diarrhea, such as with loss of body fluids and emaciation.

Bedwetting

TREATMENT PRESCRIPTION

Primary Points: Kidney (MA-SC), Bladder (MA-SC8), and Subcortex (MA-AT1).

Supplementary Points: Add Endocrine (MA-IC3) for weak constitution; add Central Rim (MA-AT) for deeper sleep; add External Genitals (MA-H4) when wet diapers or some other stimulus to the external genitals plays a role in the bed wetting.

THERAPEUTIC METHODS

Ear Acupressure: Use all the primary points together with one or two supplementary points, according to the patient's condition. Press the seeds three to five times per day, two to three minutes each time. Begin treatment on a single ear and change to the opposite ear every five to seven days.

Needle Implantation: Use all the primary points together with one or two supplementary points. Quickly insert intradermal needles into the selected points to the depth of the auricular perichondrium. Press the implanted needles three to five times per day, two to three minutes each time. Begin treatment on a single ear and change to the opposite ear every five to seven days.

CASE STUDY: BEDWETTING

According to reports, Li, a 6-year-old boy, had bedwetting every night during sleep and normally woke up after passing urine. A physical examination showed no explanation for this. The diagnosis was "enuresis."

Treatment Prescription: Kidney (MA-SC), Bladder (MA-SC8), Ear Center (MA-H1), Central Rim (MA-AT), Subcortex (MA-AT1), Endocrine (MA-IC3), and Forehead (MA-AT).

Therapeutic Method: Seed acupressure was used on one ear at a time and was switched to the other ear twice a week. The patient was instructed to press the seeds three to five times per day during the treatment.

Treatment Results: The patient was able to wake up to urinate after four treatments. A total of eight treatments were given to enhance the therapeutic results.

Comments: 1. This treatment increases cerebral cortex excitement, reduces drowsiness on awakening, and enhances urine storage of the bladder. The points for tranquilizing should be avoided.

2. Parents should support their children to ease psychological pressures. Parents can also monitor the amount of fluids consumed after lunch time, remind the child to urinate before bed time, and wake up the child to urinate at night.

Hyperactivity

TREATMENT PRESCRIPTION

Primary Points: Subcortex (MA-AT1), Kidney (MA-SC), and Heart (MA-IC).

Supplementary Points: Add Ear Shén Mén (MA-TF1) for forgetfulness and dream-disturbed sleep; add Spleen (MA-IC) for poor appetite; add Liver (MA-SC5) for shortness of temper.

THERAPEUTIC METHOD

Ear Acupressure: Use all the primary points together with one or two supplementary points, according to the patient's condition. Press the seeds three to five times per day until obvious distention, heat, and pain are felt. Begin treatment on a single ear and change to the opposite ear every five to seven days.

CASE STUDY: ATTENTION DEFICIT AND HYPERACTIVITY DISORDER (ADHD)

Xu, a 10-year-old boy, chronically suffered from poor concentration and hyperactive behavior; he got poor grades in school as a result. The diagnosis was "hyperactivity."

Treatment Prescription: Heart (MA-IC), Kidney (MA-SC), Central Rim (MA-AT), Subcortex (MA-AT1), and Forehead (MA-AT).

Therapeutic Method: Seed acupressure was applied to all the above points. The ears were treated alternately, switching ears every three days. The patient was told to press the seeds three to five times per day during the treatment.

Treatment Results: All the symptoms were remarkably improved after 10 treatments. After seed acupressure was applied for another 20 treatments, the symptoms were all relieved and his school grades were remarkably improved.

Comments: 1. This treatment is helpful for any conditions of unsettled spirit and/or physical hyperactive behavior. The diagnosis of hyperactivity, or related biomedical disorders such as ADHD, should be made by a specialist before treatment.

2. Parents and teachers should try to stay closely tuned to the child's demeanor during treatment, in order to help regulate the child's psychological state.

EYE, EAR, NOSE AND THROAT DISORDERS

Sty

TREATMENT PRESCRIPTION

Primary Points: Liver (MA-SC5), Eye (MA-L1), and Heart (MA-IC).

Supplementary Points: Add Ear Apex (MA-H6) and Adrenal Gland (MA-T) for severe redness and swelling; add Ear Shén Mén (MA-TF1) and

Subcortex (MA-AT1) for severe itching and pain; add Kidney (MA-SC) and Spleen (MA-IC) for multiple sties.

THERAPEUTIC METHODS

Bloodletting: Quickly prick with a three-edged needle at Ear Apex (MA-H6) or on the vein of the posterior surface that is closest to Ear Apex, to draw two or three drops of blood. Treat once per day. Begin treatment on a single ear and change to the opposite ear every other day until the sty is healed.

Moxibustion: Select two or three primary points together with one or two supplementary points. Begin treatment on a single ear and change to the opposite ear every other day. The moxibustion is done using medicated thread at the points. Continue moxibustion for five to ten minutes or until the patient feels a mild burning sensation. This type of moxibustion can also be used on the protuberances of the affected area to promote drainage of infected matter. Treat once per day; one treatment course is five days.

Ear Acupuncture: Select all primary points together with supplementary points, according to the patient's condition. Retain the needles 30 to 60 minutes and manipulate every 10 to 15 minutes, using strong stimulation by applying lifting and thrusting and needle rotation. Treat one or two times per day. Begin treatment on a single ear and change to the opposite ear every three to five days. One treatment course is five to seven days.

CASE STUDY: STY

Tang, a 20-year-old female, suffered from swelling and pain on the right eyelid for one day, with redness around the affected area. The diagnosis was "sty."

Treatment Prescription: A small varicose vein was selected on the upper 1/3 of the posterior surface from the ear root toward the helix.

Therapeutic Method: The selected area was sterilized; the vein was pricked from lateral side to medial, and one to three drops of blood was drawn.

Treatment Results: Eight hours after the treatment, redness and swelling was gone and the pain was relieved.

Comments: 1. This treatment can only be used for early stage of sty that is marked by redness and swelling. It is not effective for the pus formation stage.

2. If there is no bleeding from pricking the varicose vein indicated above, use a three-edged needle to bleed Ear Apex (MA-H6).

Myopia (Pseudomyopia)

TREATMENT PRESCRIPTION

Primary Points: Eye (MA-L1), Liver (MA-SC5), Kidney (MA-SC), and Occiput (MA-AT).

Supplementary Points: Add Forehead (MA-AT) and Apex of Antitragus (MA-AT) for astigmatism; add Ear Shén Mén (MA-TF1) and Adrenal Gland (MA-T) for night blindness; add Adrenal Gland (MA-T) and Subcortex (MA-AT1) for retinitis; add Heart (MA-IC), Spleen (MA-IC), and Apex of Antitragus (MA-AT) for nearsightedness.

THERAPEUTIC METHODS

Ear Acupressure: Select two or three primary points together with one or two supplementary points. Press the vaccaria seeds three to five times per day, two to three minutes each time, or until sensations of soreness, distention, pain, or heat are induced. Begin treatment on a single ear and change to the opposite ear every other day.

Ear Acupuncture: Select all primary points together with supplementary points, according to the patient's condition. Retain the needles 30 to 60 minutes and manipulate every 10 to 15 minutes using needle scratching and rotation. Treat one or two times per day. Begin treatment on a single ear and change to the opposite ear every other session. One treatment course is five to seven days; allow two or three days between treatment courses.

NOTES

• Ear acupuncture is only effective for treating pseudomyopia.

Infectious Conjunctivitis/Wind-Fire Eye

TREATMENT PRESCRIPTION

Primary Points: Eye (MA-L1), Liver (MA-SC5), Lung (MA-IC1), and Ear Apex (MA-H6).

Supplementary Points: Add Eye (MA-L1) and Endocrine (MA-IC3) for photophobia and tearing; add Forehead (MA-AT) and Ear Shén Mén (MA-TF1) for painful eyes; add Heart (MA-IC) and Adrenal Gland (MA-T) for burning sensation of eyes and swelling of eyelids.

THERAPEUTIC METHODS

Bloodletting: Prick Ear Apex (MA-H6) and the vein on the posterior surface of the auricle with a three-edged needle to draw three to five drops of blood. Treat once per day. Begin treatment on a single ear and change to the opposite ear every other day until the disorder is healed.

Ear Acupuncture: Use all the primary points together with one or two supplementary points, according to the patient's condition. Retain the needles 30 to 60 minutes and manipulate every 10 to 15 minutes, using strong stimulation by applying lifting and thrusting and needle rotation. Treat one or two times per day. Begin treatment on a single ear and change to the opposite ear every other day. One treatment course is five to seven days; allow two or three days between treatment courses. Continue treatments until the bloodshot eyes are healed.

Ear Acupressure: Select two or three primary points together with one or two supplementary points. Press the vaccaria seeds three to five times per day, two to three minutes each time. Begin treatment on a single ear and change to the opposite ear every other day.

NOTES

- In the epidemic stage of acute conjunctivitis, ear acupressure at Eye (MA-L1), Liver (MA-SC5), and Lung (MA-IC1) in both ears can prevent the eyes from becoming infected.

Ophthalmia

TREATMENT PRESCRIPTION

Primary Points: Eye (MA-L1), Liver (MA-SC5), and Adrenal Gland (MA-T).

Supplementary Points: Add Ear Shén Mén (MA-TF1) for pain and burning sensation; add Kidney (MA-SC) for chronic cases with corneal damage.

THERAPEUTIC METHODS

Ear Acupuncture: Use all the primary points together with one or both supplementary points, according to the patient's condition. Retain the needles 30 to 60 minutes and manipulate every 10 to 15 minutes, using strong stimulation by applying lifting and thrusting and needle rotation. Treat one or two times per day. Begin treatment on a single ear and change to the opposite ear every other day. One treatment course is five to seven days; allow two or three days between treatment courses. Continue treating until bloodshot eyes are healed.

Needle Implantation: Select the same points as above. Implant the intradermal needles at the selected points, then press the needles three to five times per day, two to three minutes each time. Begin treatment on a single ear and change to the opposite ear every five to seven days. In general, ophthalmia can be healed after two or three treatments.

CASE STUDY: OPHTHALMIA

Zhao, a 30-year-old male, suffered from severe pain of both eyes with severe photophobia and tearing after damage by an arc flash while welding at work. Physical examination showed hyperemia of the bulbar conjunctiva on both eyes and swelling. The diagnosis was "ophthalmia."

Treatment Prescription: Ear Apex (MA-H6), Eye (MA-L1), Liver (MA-SC5), Adrenal Gland (MA-T), Subcortex (MA-AT1), and Ear Shén Mén (MA-TF1).

Therapeutic Method: Draw one to three drops of blood at Ear Apex (MA-H6) and needle all the other points on both ears with strong stimulation; retain the needles for 30 minutes.

Treatment Results: All the symptoms were remarkably improved after the first treatment. The symptoms were entirely relieved with a total of three treatments.

Comments: 1. In the patient with congestion of the bulbar conjunctiva there is always a varicose vein on the upper 1/3 of the posterior surface of both ears. Pricking to cause bleeding on one ear brings enhanced therapeutic results.

2. Sunglasses are needed to prevent strong lights from stimulating the affected eyes during treatment.

Tonsillitis/Baby Moth

TREATMENT PRESCRIPTION

Primary Points: Tonsil (MA-L), Pharynx and Larynx (MA-T3), and Lung (MA-IC1).

Supplementary Points: Add Ear Apex (MA-H6) and Adrenal Gland (MA-T) in the acute stage; add Endocrine (MA-IC3) and Kidney (MA-SC) in the chronic stage.

Bloodletting: This method is only used for acute cases. Use a three-edged needle to prick Ear Apex (MA-H6) or the "ouch" point (ashii point) along the line connecting Ear Center (MA-H1) to Ear Apex (MA-H6). Treat once every other day until the sore throat is gone.

Ear Acupuncture: Use all the primary points together with one or two supplementary points, according to the patient's condition. Retain the needles 30 to 60 minutes and manipulate every 10 to 15 minutes, using strong stimulation by applying lifting and thrusting and needle rotation. Treat one or two times per day. Begin treatment on a single ear and change to the opposite ear every other day. One treatment course is five to seven days; allow two or three days between treatment courses.

Ear Acupressure: Select two or three primary points together with one or two supplementary points. Affix Six Spirits Pills *(Liù Shén Wán)* to strengthen the function of clearing heat and resolving toxins. Press the pills three to five times per day, three to five minutes each time. Begin treatment on a single ear and change to the opposite ear every other day.

Recurrent Mouth Ulcerations

TREATMENT PRESCRIPTION

Primary Points: Mouth (MA-IC5), Tongue (MA-L), and Endocrine (MA-IC3).

Supplementary Points: Add Stomach (MA-IC) and Large Intestine (MA-SC4) for poor appetite and constipation due to heat brewing in the spleen and stomach; add Heart (MA-IC) and Spleen (MA-IC) for heat accumulated in the Spleen and Heart; add Liver (MA-SC5) and Gallbladder (MA-SC6) for depressed heat in the liver and gallbladder; add Kidney (MA-SC) and Ear Shén Mén (MA-TF1) for breakdown of heart-kidney interaction; add *Sān Jiāo* (MA-IC4) for exuberant damp; add Ear Apex (MA-H6) for exuberant heat.

THERAPEUTIC METHODS

Ear Acupuncture: Use all the primary points together with one or two supplementary points, according to the patient's condition. Begin treatment on a single ear and change to the opposite ear every other day, using needle scratching and rotation. Retain the needles 30 minutes and manipulate every 10 minutes. Treat once per day. One treatment course is five to seven days; allow two or three days between treatment courses.

Ear Acupressure: Select two or three primary points together with one or two supplementary points. Affix Six Spirits Pills *(Liù Shén Wán)* to strengthen the function of clearing heat and resolving toxins. Press the pills three to five times per day, three to five minutes each time. Begin treatment on a single ear and change to the opposite ear every five to seven days. One treatment course is seven days.

NOTES

* Ear acupuncture can also be used to prevent recurrence of ulcerated sores in the mouth.

Toothache

TREATMENT PRESCRIPTION

Primary Points: Tooth (MA-L), Jaw (MA-L), and Ear Shén Mén (MA-TF1).

Supplementary Points: Add Lung (MA-IC1) for wind fire; add Stomach (MA-IC) for stomach fire; add Kidney (MA-SC) for vacuity fire; add Adrenal Gland (MA-T) for severe swelling and pain.

THERAPEUTIC METHODS

Ear Acupressure: Use all the primary points together with one or two supplementary points. Use borneol to clear heat and resolve toxins. Treat both ears at every treatment. Press the bits of borneol three to five times a day, three to five minutes each time. One treatment course is seven days.

Needle Implantation: Select two or three primary points together with one or two supplementary points. After sterilizing the ear, quickly implant the intradermal needles at the selected points. Press the needles forcefully three to five times per day, two to three minutes each time (or until redness and heat are induced in the auricle). Begin treatment on a single ear and change to the opposite ear every five to seven days.

Electroacupuncture: Select two primary points and one supplementary point. Insert needles into the selected points, and then connect the needles to an electroacupuncture apparatus for 30 minutes. Use the continuous wave setting at a frequency of 180 hz. Treat once per day. One treatment course is five to seven days.

Allergic Rhinitis

TREATMENT PRESCRIPTION

Primary Points: Internal Nose (MA-T), Lung (MA-IC1), and Adrenal Gland (MA-T).

Supplementary Points: Add Ear Shén Mén (MA-TF1) for severe nasal itching; add Kidney (MA-SC) and Endocrine (MA-IC3) for protracted cases; add Apex of Antitragus (MA-AT) for cough and panting in infants.

THERAPEUTIC METHODS

Ear Acupressure: Use all the primary points together with one or two supplementary points. Press the vaccaria seeds three to five times per day, three to five minutes each time. Begin treatment on a single ear and change to the opposite ear every five to seven days.

Medicine Injection: Use 1 ml (25 mg) of Phenergan. After sterilization, insert the needle to the depth of the auricular perichondrium. Inject the medicine into Internal Nose (MA-T), Lung (MA-IC1), and Adrenal Gland (MA-T), using 1 ml for each point. Inject the remainder at *Qū Chí* (LI-11, Pool at the Bend)—a body acupuncture point—on the same

side of the body. Begin treatment on a single ear and change to the opposite ear every other day. One treatment course is six days.

CASE STUDY: ALLERGIC RHINITIS

Cao, a 45-year-old male, had suffered for two years from runny nose
  when encountering cold air, particularly in winter. The diagnosis
  was "allergic rhinitis."

Treatment Prescription: Internal Ear (MA-L), Lung (MA-IC1), Adrenal Gland (MA-T), Endocrine (MA-IC3), and Wind Stream (MA-
  SF).

Therapeutic Method: Seed acupressure was applied to all the above
  points. The ears were treated alternately, switching ears twice a
  week. The patient was told to press the seeds three to five times
  per day during the treatment.

Treatment Results: The patient's runny nose was remarkably improved after two treatments. The symptoms were all relieved with
  a total of eight treatments.

Comments: 1. Ear acupuncture is effective for relieving all symptoms
  at the onset of allergic rhinitis.

  2. As for seasonal allergic rhinitis, ear acupuncture should
  be applied before the season comes to prevent an occurrence or to
  reduce the symptoms.

Nosebleed

TREATMENT PRESCRIPTION

Primary Points: Internal Nose (MA-T), Lung (MA-IC1), and Adrenal
Gland (MA-T).

Supplementary Points: Add Diaphragm (Ear Center, MA-H1) and
for sudden onset of nosebleed due to lung and stomach heat; add
Spleen (MA-IC) and Kidney (MA-SC) for chronic bleeding or
bloody nasal discharge due to vacuity fire.

THERAPEUTIC METHODS

Ear Acupuncture: Use all the primary points together with one or
two supplementary points, according to the patient's condition. Retain the
needles 30 to 60 minutes and manipulate every 10 to 15 minutes, using
moderate stimulation by applying lifting and thrusting and needle rotation. Treat one or two times per day. Begin treatment on a single ear and
change to the opposite ear every other day. One treatment course is five to
seven days; allow two or three days between treatment courses.

Ear Acupressure: Select two or three primary points together with one or two supplementary points. Press the vaccaria seeds three to five times per day, three to five minutes each time. Begin treatment on a single ear and change to the opposite ear every five to seven days.

NOTES

• Other therapies should be added for severe nosebleed.

Chronic Otitis Media

TREATMENT PRESCRIPTION

Primary Points: Internal Ear (MA-L), Ear Center (MA-H1), and Endocrine (MA-IC3).

Supplementary Points: Add Lung (MA-IC1), Pancreas/Gallbladder (MA-SC6), and Adrenal Gland (MA-T) for chronic catarrhal otitis media; add Kidney (MA-SC), Liver (MA-SC5), and *Sān Jiāo* (MA-IC4) for chronic suppurative otitis media.

THERAPEUTIC METHODS

Ear Acupressure: Use all the primary points together with one or two supplementary points. Press the vaccaria seeds three to five times per day, three to five minutes each time. Begin treatment on a single ear and change to the opposite ear every five to seven days.

Needle Implantation: Use all the primary points together with one or two supplementary points. After sterilization, implant intradermal needles at the selected points. Press the implanted needles three to five times per day, two to three minutes each time. Begin treatment on a single ear and change to the opposite ear every five to seven days.

Auditory Vertigo

TREATMENT PRESCRIPTION

Primary Points: Internal Ear (MA-L), Kidney (MA-SC), Ear Shén Mén (MA-TF1), and Occiput (MA-AT).

Supplementary Points: Add Liver (MA-SC5) and Sympathetic (MA-AH7) for severe dizziness; add Spleen (MA-IC) and Stomach (MA-IC) for severe vomiting.

THERAPEUTIC METHODS

Ear Acupuncture: Select two or three primary points together with one or two supplementary points, according to the patient's condition. Retain the needles 30 to 60 minutes and manipulate every 10 to 15 minutes, using moderate stimulation by needle rotation. Treat once per day; for severe cases, treat twice per day. Begin treatment on a single ear and change to the opposite ear every other day. One treatment course is five to seven days; allow two or three days between treatment courses.

Ear Acupressure: Select two or three primary points together with one or two supplementary points. Press the vaccaria seeds three to five times per day, three to five minutes each time. Begin treatment on a single · ear and change to the opposite ear every five to seven days.

CASE STUDY: MENIÈRE'S SYNDROME

Cui, a 42-year-old female, sought treatment after suffering from severe vertigo for one day. The vertigo occurred suddenly when she was trying to get up from bed. She also had nausea, vomiting, and an inability to turn the head and body. A few years earlier, the patient had vertigo attacks. Physical examination revealed no explanation for this problem. The diagnosis was "Menière's Syndrome."

Treatment Prescription: Internal Ear (MA-L), Kidney (MA-SC), Liver (MA-SC5), *Sān Jiāo* (MA-IC4), Subcortex (MA-AT1), Sympathetic (MA-AH7), and Ear Shén Mén (MA-TF1).

Therapeutic Method: Seed acupressure was applied to all the above points. Both ears were treated simultaneously. The patient was told to press the seeds three to five times per day during the treatment.

Treatment Results: Vertigo was improved two hours after treatment. The patient could get up from bed and move around at home after the second treatment. After the third treatment, all the symptoms were completely gone, and the therapeutic effect was stabilized.

Comments: 1. Ear acupuncture can relieve all the symptoms for Menière's Syndrome whenever it occurs. But it cannot completely heal the patient.

2. This therapy is ineffective for vertigo due to misuse of medicines, such as streptomycin.

SKIN DISEASES

Urticaria

TREATMENT PRESCRIPTION

Primary Points: Wind Stream (MA-SF), Lung (MA-IC1), Adrenal Gland (MA-T) and Endocrine (MA-IC3).

Supplementary Points: Add Spleen (MA-IC) and Stomach (MA-IC) for nausea and vomiting; add Large Intestine (MA-SC4) for constipation; add Ear Shén Mén (MA-TF1) for irritability.

THERAPEUTIC METHODS

Ear Acupressure: Use all the primary points together with one or two supplementary points. Press the vaccaria seeds three to five times per day, or whenever itching occurs; continue pressing for three to five minutes each time. Begin treatment on a single ear and change to the opposite ear every five to seven days.

Needle Implantation: Use all the primary points together with one or two supplementary points. After sterilization, implant intradermal needles at the selected points. Press the implanted needles three to five times per day, two to three minutes each time. Begin treatment on a single ear and change to the opposite ear every five to seven days.

CASE STUDY: URTICARIA

Lu, a 40-year-old male, suffered from severe skin itching one hour after eating sea food. Physical examination showed red skin rashes and pale red patches all over the trunk and limbs. The diagnosis was "urticaria."

Treatment Prescription: Ear Apex (MA-H6), Lung (MA-IC1), Liver (MA-SC5), Spleen (MA-IC), Endocrine (MA-IC3), Subcortex (MA-AT1), Sympathetic (MA-AH7), Adrenal Gland (MA-T), Wind Stream (MA-SF), and Ear Shén Mén (MA-TF1).

Therapeutic Method: Bleed one to three drops of blood at Ear Apex (MA-H6); needle all other points on both ears with strong stimulation, and retain the needles for 30 minutes.

Treatment Results: Skin redness and itching were remarkably improved after 10 minutes of treatment. Skin rashes started to be reduced six hours later.

Comment:

The above therapy is effective for acute urticaria. It does not provide satisfying treatment results for chronic conditions, particularly for patients on hormone treatment.

Eczema

TREATMENT PRESCRIPTION

Primary Points: Lung (MA-IC1), Adrenal Gland (MA-T), Endocrine (MA-IC3), and Wind Stream (MA-SF).

Supplementary Points: Add Occiput (MA-AT) for severe itching of skin; add Ear Shén Mén (MA-TF1) and Heart (MA-IC) for irritability; add Spleen (MA-IC) and Sympathetic (MA-AH7) for oozing skin lesions; add Large Intestine (MA-SC4) and Pancreas/Gallbladder (MA-SC6) for constipation and bitter taste in the mouth.

THERAPEUTIC METHODS

Ear Acupuncture: Use all the primary points together with one or two supplementary points, according to the patient's condition. Retain the needles 60 minutes and manipulate every 10 to 15 minutes, using moderate stimulation by needle scratching and rotation. Treat once per day. Begin treatment on a single ear and change to the opposite ear every other day. One treatment course is five to seven days; allow two or three days between treatment courses.

Ear Acupressure: This method is especially effective for chronic eczema. Select two or three primary points together with one or two supplementary points. Use mung beans. Press the beans three to five times per day, three to five minutes each time. Begin treatment on a single ear and change to the opposite ear every five to seven days.

Bloodletting: This method is used to treat acute eczema with fever or for protracted cases. Bloodletting is done in the small veins on the posterior surface of the ear, drawing two or three drops of blood each time. Treatment is done one time per day.

Neurodermatitis

TREATMENT PRESCRIPTION

Primary Points: Liver (MA-SC5), Lung (MA-IC1), and Adrenal Gland (MA-T).

Supplementary Points: Add Occiput (MA-AT) and Parotid Gland (MA-AT) for severe itching; add Heart (MA-IC) and Ear Shén Mén (MA-TF1) for vexation and insomnia; add Spleen (MA-IC) and Endocrine (MA-IC3) for redness, erosion, and wet ulcers in affected areas.

THERAPEUTIC METHODS

Bloodletting (at Points): Select two primary points together with one supplementary point. After sterilization, cut a 2 to 3 mm opening with a surgical blade at each selected point until blood or tissue fluid flows out, then bandage the wound. Treat one or two times per week. Begin treatment on a single ear and change to the opposite ear every other session. One treatment course is five treatments.

Bloodletting (on the Posterior Surface): Prick the veins in the upper, middle, and lower parts of the posterior surface of the ear with a three-edged needle to draw 1-3 ml of blood. Treat once every three days. Begin treatment on a single ear and change to the opposite ear every other session. One treatment course is six treatments.

Medicine Injection: Select one or two primary points together with one supplementary point. Prepare 2 ml (100mg) of vitamin C, using 0.1 ml for each point. The rest is injected into *Qū Chí* (LI-11, Pool at the Bend). Treat once per day. Begin treatment on a single ear and change to the opposite ear every other day. One treatment course is seven treatments.

Pruritus

TREATMENT PRESCRIPTION

Primary Points: Lung (MA-IC1), Adrenal Gland (MA-T), and Endocrine (MA-IC3).

Supplementary Points: Add Liver (MA-SC5) and Kidney (MA-SC) for older adults due to blood vacuity engendering dryness. Add Pancreas/Gallbladder (MA-SC6) and Large Intestine (MA-SC4) for bitter taste and constipation due to damp-heat; add Ear Shén Mén (MA-TF1) for insomnia; add Pancreas/Gallbladder (MA-SC6) when pruritus is associated with diabetes.

THERAPEUTIC METHODS

Ear Acupressure: Select two or three primary points together with one or two supplementary points. Press the vaccaria seeds three to five times per day, three to five minutes each time (or until numbness and distention are felt in the auricle). Begin treatment on a single ear and change to the opposite ear every five to seven days.

Needle Implantation: Use all the primary points together with one or two supplementary points. After sterilization, implant intradermal needles at the selected points. Press the needles four or five times per day, one to two minutes each time. Begin treatment on a single ear and change to the opposite ear every five to seven days.

CASE STUDY: ITCHING SKIN

Song, a 68-year-old female, had suffered for the last six months from itching skin that was worse at night and accompanied by insomnia. Physical examination showed dry, scratched skin with skin damage due to scratching.

Treatment Prescription: Ear Apex (MA-H6), Liver (MA-SC5), Spleen (MA-IC), Lung (MA-IC1), Endocrine (MA-IC3), Wind Stream (MA-SF), Occiput (MA-AT), and Ear Center (MA-H1).

Therapeutic Method: Bleed one to three drops of blood at Ear Apex (MA-H6); apply seed acupressure to all other points. The ears were treated alternately, switching ears twice a week. The patient was told to press the seeds three to four times per day, plus one more time 30 minutes before bedtime.

> **Treatment Results:** Itching was remarkably improved after four treatments. The symptoms were all relieved after a total of eight treatments. Another four treatments were given to strengthen the therapeutic effect.
>
> **Comments:** 1. Ear acupuncture is effective for quick relief of itching, but does not remove the caus. Thus, a treatment for the pathogen is needed in addition to ear acupuncture.
>
>   2. For a reliable therapeutic result, continue seed acupressure for one month after all the symptoms are gone.

Herpes Zoster

TREATMENT PRESCRIPTION

Primary Points: Liver (MA-SC5), Pancreas/Gallbladder (MA-SC6), and Ear Shén Mén (MA-TF1).

Supplementary Points: Add Subcortex (MA-AT1) and Sympathetic (MA-AH7) for severe pain; add Spleen (MA-IC) and Lung (MA-IC1) for skin lesions with erosion and wet ulcers.

THERAPEUTIC METHODS

Ear Acupressure: Select one or two primary points together with one supplementary point. Use 0.2 to 0.3 cm borneol. Press, knead, and pinch the borneol pieces three to five times per day, and continue pressing until numbness, pain, and a burning sensation are felt in the auricle. Treat both ears simultaneously.

Ear Acupuncture: Select two or three primary points together with one or two supplementary points, according to the patient's condition. Retain the needles 30 minutes and manipulate every 10 minutes, using moderate stimulation by needle scratching and rotation. Treat once per day. Begin treatment on a single ear and change to the opposite ear every other day. Continue treatment until the herpes zoster is gone and pain is relieved.

Radiation Therapy: Use a helium-neon laser apparatus. Position the transmitting probe 10 to 20 mm from the selected points. Irradiate each point for two minutes. Treat once per day. Begin treatment on a single ear and change to the opposite ear every other day. One treatment course is ten days.

NOTES

- Borneol clears head and relieves pain.
- When borneol is absorbed by the skin, it strengthens the therapeutic effect.

- Protective glasses are needed for the practitioner during treatments when a laser is used.

Leukoderma

TREATMENT PRESCRIPTION

Primary Points: Sympathetic (MA-AH7), Endocrine (MA-IC3), Lung (MA-IC1), and Diaphragm (Ear Center, MA-H1).

Supplementary Points: Add Adrenal Gland (MA-T) and Ear Shén Mén (MA-TF1) for neurodermatitis; add Heart (MA-IC) and Occiput (MA-AT) for alopecia areata; add Forehead (MA-AT) and Brain (MA-AT) for lesions about the face and head; add corresponding points for lesions occurring on the dorsum of the hands, the extremities, or the trunk.

THERAPEUTIC METHODS

Ear Acupressure: Select two or three primary points together with one or two supplementary points. Use rapeseeds in larger sizes. Press, knead, and pinch the seeds three to five times per day, gradually increasing the intensity and frequency of the pressing. In general, milder manipulations are used for vacuity patterns, and stronger ones for repletion patterns. Begin treatment on a single ear and change to the opposite ear every five to seven days.

Needle Implantation: Use all the primary points together with one or two supplementary points. After sterilization, implant intradermal needles at the selected points. Press the needles three to five times per day, two to three minutes each time. Begin treatment on a single ear and change to the opposite ear every five to seven days.

CASE STUDY: LEUKODERMA

Yu, a 20-year-old female, complained of two patches of discoloration that had been on her body for the last year. One was on the left ankle, the other on the chest. Both of the patches were 2 X 3 cm. Another discolored patch had appeared two months prior on the lateral end of the left eyebrow. There was no abnormal sensation on the affected skin areas. The diagnosis was "leukoderma."

Treatment Prescription: Ear Apex (MA-H6), Forehead (MA-AT), Lung (MA-IC1), Kidney (MA-SC), Adrenal Gland (MA-T), Central Rim (MA-AT), Endocrine (MA-IC3), Subcortex (MA-AT1), and Wind Stream (MA-SF).

Therapeutic Method: Bleeding at Ear Apex (MA-H6); seed acupressure for all other points. The ears were alternately treated, switching ears twice a week. The patient was told to press the seeds three to five times per day during the treatment.

Treatment Results: The white patch on the forehead turned red after 10 treatments. Black spots covered over the affected area after four treatments. The skin color returned normal after a total of eight treatments. The two other patches on the chest and ankle gradually returned to normal after one year of treatment.

Comments: 1. Ear acupuncture treatment can significantly slow down the development of leukoderma. Early treatment in younger patients is always followed by better therapeutic results.

2. Ear acupuncture treatment requires a long treatment course; the patient should have patience in waiting for the results.

3. Considering that the occurrence of leukoderma can be related to a lack of certain trace elements, ear acupuncture is more effective when accompanied with vitamin/trace element therapy.

Psoriasis

TREATMENT PRESCRIPTION

Primary Points: Lung (MA-IC1), Endocrine (MA-IC3), Ear Apex (MA-H6) and corresponding areas.

Supplementary Points: Add Heart (MA-IC)´ and Ear Shén Mén (MA-TF1) for severe itching that disturbs sleep; add Liver (MA-SC5) and Kidney (MA-SC) for profuse scales; add Large Intestine (MA-SC4) and Occiput (MA-AT) for bright red skin lesions, constipation, and foul breath.

THERAPEUTIC METHODS

Ear Acupuncture: Insert a filiform needle from Ear Apex (MA-H6) along the subcutaneous layer to the root of the ear, then rotate the needle for five minutes. Insert needles into the other points as deep as the auricular perichondrium. Retain 30 minutes after needle rotation, and manipulate every 10 minutes. Treat once per day. Begin treatment on a single ear and change to the opposite ear every other day. One treatment course is seven to ten days; allow two or three days between treatment courses.

Point-cutting: Select two or three primary points together with one or two supplementary points. Cut a one to two mm opening at the points with a surgical blade to draw blood, and then apply ointment mixed with garlic and pepper paste. Treat once every three days. Begin treatment on a single ear and change to the opposite ear every other session. One treatment course is one month.

Bloodletting: Prick with a three-edged needle at Ear Apex (MA-H6) and other corresponding points to draw three to five drops of blood. Treat one time every other day. Begin treatment on a single ear and change to the opposite ear every other session. One treatment course is ten treatments.

Flat Wart

TREATMENT PRESCRIPTION

Primary Points: Lung (MA-IC1), Endocrine (MA-IC3), Subcortex (MA-AT1), and other corresponding points.

Supplementary Points: Kidney (MA-SC), Heart (MA-IC), Adrenal Gland (MA-T), Ear Shén Mén (MA-TF1), and Posterior Surface (MA-PS).

THERAPEUTIC METHODS

Needle Implantation: Select two or three primary points together with one or two supplementary points. After sterilization, implant intradermal needles at the selected points. Press the implanted needles three to five times per day, two to three minutes each time. Begin treatment on a single ear and change to the opposite ear every five to seven days.

Radiation Therapy: Use a helium-neon laser apparatus. Position the transmitting probe 10 to 20 mm from the selected points. Irradiate each point for two minutes. Treat once per day. Begin treatment on a single ear and change to the opposite ear every other day. One treatment course is ten treatments.

Bloodletting: Select the internal boundary of Groove of Posterior Surface (MA-PS). Prick the small veins at the upper, middle, and lower parts of the posterior surface to draw five to ten drops of blood. Treat two times per week. Begin treatment on a single ear and change to the opposite ear at the next treatment session. One treatment course is ten treatments.

Erythromelalgia

TREATMENT PRESCRIPTION

Primary Points: Sympathetic (MA-AH7), Ear Shén Mén (MA-TF1), and Heart (MA-IC).

Supplementary Points: Subcortex (MA-AT1) and corresponding points.

THERAPEUTIC METHODS

Electroacupuncture: Select two or three primary points together with one or two supplementary points, according to the patient's condition. Insert needles into the selected points and connect them to an electroacupuncture apparatus set at pulsating current (alternating between strong and weak) for 30 to 60 minutes. Treat one or two times per day.

Begin treatment on a single ear and change to the opposite ear every other day. One treatment course is five to seven days. Continue treating once per day after symptoms are relieved.

Ear Acupressure: All points are used. Press the vaccaria seeds three to five times per day or whenever severe pain occurs. Continue pressing for two to three minutes each time, or until the pain is relieved. Begin treatment on a single ear and change to the opposite ear every five to seven days. One treatment course is five to seven days; allow two or three days between treatment courses.

PREVENTIVE THERAPY AND BEAUTY ENHANCEMENT

Prevention of the Common Cold

TREATMENT PRESCRIPTION

Primary Points: External Nose (MA-T1), Pharynx and Larynx (MA-T3), Lung (MA-IC1), and Kidney (MA-SC).

Supplementary Points: Ear Apex (MA-H6), Occiput (MA-AT), Adrenal Gland (MA-T), Spleen (MA-IC), Endocrine (MA-IC3), and Large Intestine (MA-SC4).

THERAPEUTIC METHODS

Point massage: Depending upon the patient's condition, knead while pressing both tragi with fingers, or knead while pressing the prescribed points with a stick to disperse the exterior and promote lung qì. Also, knead while pressing External Nose (MA-T1), Lung (MA-IC1), Pharynx and Larynx (MA-T3), and Kidney (MA-SC) with the thumb and index finger in opposition. Continue kneading 10 to 30 times for each point; treat three times per day. Begin treatment on a single ear and change to the opposite ear every other day.

Ear Acupressure: Select two or three primary points together with one or two supplementary points. Press the vaccaria seeds three to five times per day, two to three minutes each time. Begin treatment on a single ear and change to the opposite ear every five to seven days.

Smoking Cessation

TREATMENT PRESCRIPTION 1

Primary Points: Lung (MA-IC1), Stomach (MA-IC), and Ear Shén Mén (MA-TF1).

Supplementary Points: Endocrine (MA-IC3), Subcortex (MA-AT1), and Adrenal Gland (MA-T).

THERAPEUTIC METHOD

Needle Implantation: Use all the primary points together with one or two supplementary points. After sterilization, implant needles at sensitive spots in the selected areas, then fix them with an adhesive bandage. Press the needles three to five times per day, two to three minutes each time. Begin treatment on a single ear and change to the opposite ear every five to seven days.

Ear Acupressure: Select two or three primary points together with one or two supplementary points. Press the vaccaria seeds three to five times per day, two to three minutes each time (or until the desire to smoke disappears). Begin treatment on a single ear and change to the opposite ear every five to seven days.

TREATMENT PRESCRIPTION 2

Primary Points: Mouth (MA-IC5), Lung (MA-IC1), and Ear Shén Mén (MA-TF1).

Supplementary Points: Liver (MA-SC5), Subcortex (MA-AT1), Endocrine (MA-IC3), and Stomach (MA-IC).

THERAPEUTIC METHOD

Radiation Therapy: Select two or three primary points together with one or two supplementary points. Using a helium-neon laser apparatus, position the transmitting probe 10 to 20 mm from the selected points. Irradiate each point for three to five minutes. Treat once per day. Begin treatment on a single ear and change to the opposite ear every other day. One treatment course is five to seven days.

NOTES

- Ear acupuncture has proved to be significantly effective as an aid in giving up smoking tobacco. Most people feel that the taste of tobacco changes in a way that decreases their desire to smoke during the treatment period.
- Recent research indicates ear acupuncture may engender an endogenous, morphine-like substance that controls the desire to smoke and eliminates tobacco cessation symptoms.
- Confidence and determination are the most important factors for success in giving up smoking.

Alcohol Cessation

TREATMENT PRESCRIPTION

Primary Points: Ear Shén Mén (MA-TF1), Subcortex (MA-AT1), and Endocrine (MA-IC3). Clinically an additional point, Drunkenness Point (MA-SC2), located between Kidney and Small Intestine, is used.[17]

Supplementary Points: Heart (MA-IC), Stomach (MA-IC), Liver (MA-SC5), Mouth (MA-IC5), Occiput (MA-AT), Central Rim (MA-AT), and Sympathetic (MA-AH7).

THERAPEUTIC METHODS

Needle Implantation: After sterilization, select two or three primary points together with one or two supplementary points. Implant needles at the selected points and affix them with an adhesive bandage. Press the implanted needles three to five times per day, two to three minutes each time. Also press the needles when encountering the desire to drink, until that desire stops. Begin treatment on a single ear and change to the opposite ear every five to seven days.

Ear Acupressure: Select two or three primary points together with one or two supplementary points. Press the vaccaria seeds three to five times per day, two to three minutes each time, or until the desire to drink alcohol disappears. Begin treatment on a single ear and change to the opposite ear every other day.

Substance Withdrawal Syndrome

CLINICAL NOTES

Substance withdrawal syndrome refers to listlessness, restlessness, dizziness, headache, nausea, drooling, and/or general discomfort throughout the body resulting from cessation of substances such as nicotine, alcohol, and drugs. These symptoms can be relieved to an extent if one resumes smoking, drinking, or taking drugs again.

TREATMENT PRESCRIPTION

Primary Points: Ear Shén Mén (MA-TF1), Subcortex (MA-AT1), Lung (MA-IC1), and Endocrine (MA-IC3).

Supplementary Points: Sympathetic (MA-AH7), Stomach (MA-IC), Mouth (MA-IC5), Liver (MA-SC5), Heart (MA-IC), and Adrenal Gland (MA-T).

---

[17] See Figure 2.13, page 42.

THERAPEUTIC METHODS

Needle Implantation: Select two or three primary points together with one or two supplementary points. After sterilization, implant needles at the selected points and fix them with an adhesive bandage. Press the needles three to five times per day, two to three minutes each time; also press the needles whenever encountering a substance craving. Begin treatment on a single ear and change to the opposite ear every five to seven days.

Ear Acupressure: Select two or three primary points together with one or two supplementary points. Press the vaccaria seeds three to five times per day, two to three minutes each time, or until substance craving disappears. Begin treatment on a single ear and change to the opposite ear every five to seven days.

NOTES

- The duration for needle implantation should be longer in winter — changing to the opposite ear every five to seven days. It should be shorter in summer — changing to the opposite ear every three to five days — to prevent ears from becoming infected.

Obesity

TREATMENT PRESCRIPTION 1

Primary Points: Spleen (MA-IC), Stomach (MA-IC), Lung (MA-IC1), and *Sān Jiāo* (MA-IC4).

Supplementary Points: Endocrine (MA-IC3), Ear Shén Mén (MA-TF1), Mouth (MA-IC5), Subcortex (MA-AT1), Adrenal Gland (MA-T), and Kidney (MA-SC).

THERAPEUTIC METHOD

Ear Acupressure: Select two or three primary points together with one or two supplementary points. Use vaccaria seeds or mung beans. Press the seeds or beans three to five times per day, before each meal and at bedtime, for three to five minutes each time. Begin treatment on a single ear and change to the opposite ear every other day.

TREATMENT PRESCRIPTION 2

Primary Points: Kidney (MA-SC).

Supplementary Points: Mouth (MA-IC5), Spleen (MA-IC), Esophagus (MA-IC6), Endocrine (MA-IC3), and Subcortex (MA-AT1).

THERAPEUTIC METHOD

Medicine Injection: Kidney (MA-SC) is used together with one or two supplementary points, according to the patient's condition. Inject 0.5 ml of normal saline, vitamin B_{12}, or vitamin B_1 into each point.

Needle Implantation: Select two or three primary points together with one or two supplementary points. Implant needles at the selected points after sterilization, and then fix them with an adhesive bandage. Press the needles three to five times per day, before each meal and at bedtime, for three to five minutes each time. Begin treatment on a single ear and change to the opposite ear every five to seven days.

NOTES

- Ear acupuncture has a specific effect for treating obesity. In general, the patient will feel full and not want to eat.

- In addition to treatment, the patient should have a proper diet, including low calorie foods in small amounts, and get plenty of exercise.

Motion Sickness

Primary Points: Subcortex (MA-AT1), Ear Shén Mén (MA-TF1), and Occiput (MA-AT).

Supplementary Points: Heart (MA-IC), Stomach (MA-IC), Wind Stream (MA-SF), and External Ear (MA-T).

THERAPEUTIC METHOD

Ear Acupressure: Select one or two primary points together with one or two supplementary points. Press the vaccaria seeds for 30 to 60 minutes prior to traveling by car, ship, or plane and also during the trip. Treat both ears simultaneously.

CASE STUDY: MOTION SICKNESS

Sun, a 42-year-old female, suffered from motion sickness whenever she rode on a bus. The main manifestations were sudden paleness of face, cold sweats, nausea, and vomiting.

Treatment Prescription: Mouth (MA-IC5), Cardiac (MA-IC7), Occiput (MA-AT), Subcortex (MA-AT1), and Wind Stream (MA-SF).

Therapeutic Method: Seed acupressure was applied to all the points. Both ears were treated simultaneously with strong stimulation.

Treatment Results: All the symptoms had improved 3 minutes after treatment. The patient was told to press the seeds for another 5 minutes. The symptoms were all relieved.

Comments: 1. For mild cases, the above ear acupressure is used for Mouth (MA-IC5) on both ears. All the symptoms will be gone after pressing the seeds for 3 minutes.

2. The above therapy can also be used for prevention of motion sickness.

Prevention and Treatment of Transfusion Reaction

TREATMENT PRESCRIPTION

Primary Points: Ear Shén Mén (MA-TF1), Adrenal Gland (MA-T), and Subcortex (MA-AT1).

THERAPEUTIC METHOD

Ear Acupuncture: Treat both ears simultaneously. Use strong stimulation by applying lifting and thrusting and needle rotation. Manipulation should be continued until body temperature is reduced and other symptoms are relieved. Retain the needles for 30 to 60 minutes and manipulate every 10 to 15 minutes.

Drug Reaction

TREATMENT PRESCRIPTION

Primary Points: Adrenal Gland (MA-T), Ear Shén Mén (MA-TF1), and Subcortex (MA-AT1).

Supplementary Points: Stomach (MA-IC), Kidney (MA-SC), Heart (MA-IC), Sympathetic (MA-AH7), Ear Apex (MA-H6), Forehead (MA-AT), and Occiput (MA-AT).

THERAPEUTIC METHODS

Ear Acupuncture: Use all the primary points together with one or two supplementary points. For example, add Ear Apex (MA-H6) for fever; add Stomach (MA-IC) for nausea and vomiting; add Heart (MA-IC) and Kidney (MA-SC) for dizziness and insomnia. Moderate manipulations, such as needle scratching or rotation, should be used for patients with a weak constitution, while strong stimulation by lifting and thrusting and needle rotation should be used for patients with a strong constitution and/or mild reaction. Retain the needles for 30 to 60 minutes and manipulate every 10 to 15 minutes. Treat once per day. Begin treatment on a single ear and change to the opposite ear every other day. Continue treatment until all symptoms are relieved.

Ear Acupressure: Use all the primary points together with one or two supplementary points. Press the vaccaria seeds three to five times per day, two to three minutes each time. Begin treatment on a single ear and change to the opposite ear every five to seven days (one treatment course); allow two or three days between treatment courses.

Acne

TREATMENT PRESCRIPTION 1

Primary Points: Lung (MA-IC1), Stomach (MA-IC), Endocrine (MA-IC3), and corresponding points of the affected parts.

Supplementary Points: Adrenal Gland (MA-T), Subcortex (MA-AT1), Ear Shén Mén (MA-TF1), Spleen (MA-IC), *Sān Jiāo* (MA-IC4), and Cheek (MA-L).

THERAPEUTIC METHODS

Ear Acupuncture: Use all the primary points together with one or two supplementary points. Retain the needles 30 to 60 minutes and manipulate every 10 to 15 minutes, using needle scratching and rotation. Treat once per day. Begin treatment on a single ear and change to the opposite ear every other day. One treatment course is seven to ten days; allow two or three days between treatment courses.

Ear Acupressure: Use all the primary points together with one or two supplementary points. Press the vaccaria seeds three to five times per day, two to three minutes each time. Begin treatment on a single ear and change to the opposite ear every five to seven days (one treatment course). Allow two or three days between treatment courses.

TREATMENT PRESCRIPTION 2

Primary Points: Area below auricular apex.

THERAPEUTIC METHOD

Point-cutting: Sterilize the skin and cut a 3- 5mm opening with a surgical blade; apply a medicated paste made from 5g zanthoxylum, 20g garlic, some salt, and some ginger that has been pounded into a pulp. Change the paste every seven days. 30g coix (*yì yǐ rén),* 20g dandelion (*pǔ gōng yīng),* and 20g Yedo violet (*zǐ huā dì dīng)* may be added for severe cases. Add 10g of rhubarb root (*dà huáng)* for follicular acne.

TREATMENT PRESCRIPTION 2

Primary Points: Veins on posterior surface of both ears.

THERAPEUTIC METHOD

Bloodletting: Choose an appropriate vein and rub while kneading to produce congestion. Then prick the vein with a three-edged needle to draw five to ten drops of blood. Bloodletting is a supplementary treatment and may be added once in each course of treatment by another method. The treatment can be repeated after seven days if the acne is not healed. In general, acne will be gone after three treatments.

NOTES

- Ear acupuncture has a definite therapeutic effect on acne.

- Stimulating food such as pungent or hot food and alcohol should be avoided. Fatty food and meals rich in sugar should also be avoided. Ear acupuncture for acne also improves digestion and relieves constipation.
- Keep skin clean to reduce secretions and the accumulation of sebum.
- Acne should not be picked at, as this could lead to infection.

CASE STUDY: ACNE

Zha, an 18-year-old female, reported that for the last two years she had experienced outbreaks of boils on her forehead, both cheeks, and back. The boils were the size of mung beans or soybeans and oozed white sticky liquid when squeezed to break. When the acne healed, scars were left. The acne was worse during her menstrual period. The diagnosis was "acne."

Treatment Prescription: Ear Apex (MA-H6), Cheek (MA-L), Lung (MA-IC1), Kidney (MA-SC), Adrenal Gland (MA-T), and Endocrine (MA-IC3).

Therapeutic Method: Bleeding at Ear Apex (MA-H6) with three-edged needle; bleeding at Cheek (MA-L) with a lancet; seed acupressure for the other points. The ears were treated alternately, switching ears twice a week. The patient was told to press the seeds three to five times per day during the treatment.

Treatment Results: New outbreaks were remarkably reduced after four treatments. Redness, swelling, and hardness on the existing acne started to improve. All skin lesions were gone after eight treatments. To enhance the therapeutic result, seed acupressure was performed at all the above points every month, three days before her period, for a half year.

Comments: 1. Acne is a recurrent disorder so a long treatment course is usually needed.

2. Keep the face cleansed with a neutral (pH ~ 7.0) soap.

3. Maintaining healthy bowel movements is helpful for reducing outbreaks of acne.

Liver Spots

TREATMENT PRESCRIPTION 1

Primary Points: Liver (MA-SC5), Endocrine (MA-IC3), Lung (MA-IC1), and Cheek (MA-L).

Supplementary Points: Kidney (MA-SC), Spleen (MA-IC), Stomach (MA-IC), Heart (MA-IC), and Internal Reproductive Organs (MA-TF).

THERAPEUTIC METHODS

Ear Acupuncture: Use all the primary points together with one or two supplementary points. For example, add Internal Reproductive Organs (MA-TF) for menstrual disorders; add Kidney (MA-SC) and Liver (MA- SC5) for vacuity of liver and kidney yīn; add Heart (MA-IC) for qì vacuity complicated by blood stasis. Retain the needles 30 minutes and manipulate every 15 minutes, using needle scratching and rotation. Treat once per day. Begin treatment on a single ear and change to the opposite ear every other day. One treatment course is seven to ten days; allow two or three days between each treatment course.

Ear Acupressure: Use all the primary points together with one or two supplementary points. Press the vaccaria seeds three to five times per day, two to three minutes each time. Begin treatment on a single ear and change to the opposite ear every five to seven days (one treatment course). Allow two or three days between treatment courses.

TREATMENT PRESCRIPTION 2

Primary Points: Hot (MA-AH), Boil (MA-AH), and Subcortex (MA-AT1).

Supplementary Points: Endocrine (MA-IC3), Spleen (MA-IC), and Stomach (MA-IC).

THERAPEUTIC METHOD

Bloodletting: Prick with a three-edged needle at one of the prescribed points, once per day. Alternate among all the points during the course of treatment. Treat two times per week. Begin treatment on a single ear and change to the opposite ear every other session. One treatment course is seven days; allow two or three days between treatment courses.

NOTES

- Ear acupuncture is very effective for treating liver spots because it can reduce pigmentation.
- Hot (MA-AH) is a hot point that can be palpated in the inferior root of the antihelix on the line between Chest and Abdomen (see Figure 2.8, page 30). Treating it promotes the circulation of blood and warms yáng, and courses and frees the channels and network vessels. Boil (MA-AH) is an empirical point that would be visible on the inferior root of the antihelix on the line between Chest and Neck (see Figure 2.8, page 30). Treating it clears heat and resolves toxins, removes damp, and frees the network vessels.
- This dermal disorder may also be externally treated with poria powder one or two times a day.

CASE STUDY: HYPERPIGMENTATION

Zhou, a 34-year-old female, reported that for a long time she had but-
terfly-like skin with color change on both cheeks, and dark color
on her nose. It started when she took birth control pills. Sunlight
damaged the affected skin easily. She was in good health and had
no other complaints. The diagnosis was "hyperpigmentation."

Treatment Prescription: Cheek (MA-L), Liver (MA-SC5), Kidney
(MA-SC), Central Rim (MA-AT), Adrenal Gland (MA-T), and Endocrine (MA-IC3).

Therapeutic Method: Bleeding at Cheek (MA-L) with a lancet; seed
acupressure for the other points. The ears were treated alternately,
switching ears twice a week. The patient was told to press the
seeds three to five times per day during the treatment.

Treatment Results: After four treatments, the hyperpigmentation was
lighter in color and reduced in size. The butterfly-skin lesion was
reduced to several small patches with lighter color after six treatments. The skin color was almost normal after eight treatments.
To enhance the therapeutic result, another eight treatments were
given.

Comments: 1. For this disorder, as much as one to three months of
treatment is needed because the way to heal hyperpigmentation is
through regulating the hormone system.

2. During treatment, avoid exposure to sun or use sun-
screen to protect the skin from UVA/UVB rays.

Brandy Nose

TREATMENT PRESCRIPTION 1

Primary Points: Lung (MA-IC1), Internal Nose (MA-T), and Endocrine
(MA-IC3).

Supplementary Points: External Nose (MA-T1), Adrenal Gland
(MA-T), Ear Apex (MA-H6), and Ear Shén Mén (MA-TF1).

THERAPEUTIC METHOD

Ear Acupuncture: Use all the primary points together with one or
two supplementary points. Retain the needles 30 minutes and manipulate
every 10 minutes, using needle scratching and rotation. Treat once per
day. Begin treatment on a single ear and change to the opposite ear every
other day. One treatment course is seven to ten days; allow two or three
days between treatment courses.

TREATMENT PRESCRIPTION 2

Primary Points: Ear root.

THERAPEUTIC METHOD

Medicine Injection: Using 2–4 ml of vitamin B$_6$ or normal saline, inject from the front of the ear and along the ear root to the back of the ear in a circle. Treat once every other day. Begin treatment on a single ear and change to the opposite ear at the next treatment session. One treatment course is five to seven days.

Promoting Longevity and Slowing Aging

TREATMENT PRESCRIPTION 1

Primary Points: Kidney (MA-SC), Heart (MA-IC), Spleen (MA-IC), and Stomach (MA-IC).

Supplementary Points: Subcortex (MA-AT1), Sympathetic (MA-AH7), Ear Shén Mén (MA-TF1), Lung (MA-IC1), Liver (MA-SC5), Endocrine (MA-IC3), Large Intestine (MA-SC4), and Small Intestine (MA-SC2).

THERAPEUTIC METHOD

Ear Acupressure: Use all the primary points together with one or two supplementary points. For example, add Subcortex (MA-AT1) and Ear Shén Mén (MA-TF1) for retardation of cerebral nerve functions; add Endocrine for retardation of endocrine functions; add Liver (MA-SC5) and Sympathetic (MA-AH7) for climacteric syndrome. Press the vaccaria seeds three to five times per day, two to three minutes each time. Begin treatment on a single ear and change to the opposite ear every five to seven days (one treatment course). Allow two or three days between treatment courses.

TREATMENT PRESCRIPTION 2

Primary Points: Auricle.

THERAPEUTIC METHOD

Ear Massage: Knead both ears once a day for three to five minutes.

NOTES

- Research indicates that ear acupuncture regulates the internal environment of cells by regulating the functions of cells, promoting and balancing the metabolism of various enzymes in cells, and promoting metabolism of enzymes and composition of cells. It can also strengthen the function of the hypophysis-adrenal cortex to regulate endocrine disorders and retard slowing of adrenal gland functions, as well as increase and strengthen immune functions of T-cells. These can all be considered anti-aging effects.

- See Chapter Four for more information on auricular massage.

APPENDIX I

H1	Helix 1	lún yī	轮1
H2	Helix 2	lún èr	轮2
H3	Helix 3	lún sān	轮3
H4	Helix 4	lún sì	轮4
H5	Helix 5	lún wǔ	轮5
H6	Helix 6	lún lìu	轮6
MA-H	Liver Yáng	gān yáng	肝阳
MA-H1	Diaphragm (Ear Center)	gé (ěr zhōng)	膈
MA-H1	Ear Center (Diaphragm)	ěr zhōng (gé)	耳中
MA-H2	Rectum	zhí cháng	直肠
MA-H3	Urethra	niào dào	尿道
MA-H4	External Genitals	wài shēng zhí qì	外生殖器
MA-H5	Anus	gāng mén	肛门
MA-H6	Ear Apex	ěr jiān	耳尖
MA-SF	Rheumatic Line	fēng shī xiàn	风湿线
MA-SF	Wind Stream	fēng xī	风溪
MA-SF1	Finger	zhǐ	指
MA-SF2	Wrist	wàn	腕
MA-SF3	Elbow	zhǒu	肘
MA-SF4	Shoulder	jiān	肩
MA-SF5	Clavicle	suǒ gǔ	锁骨
MA-AH	Boil	jiē diǎn	疖点

MA-AH	Hot	rè diǎn	热点
MA-AH	Toe	zú zhǐ	足趾
MA-AH1	Heel	gēn	跟
MA-AH2	Ankle	huái	踝
MA-AH3	Knee	xī	膝
MA-AH4	Hip	kuān	髋
MA-AH5	Buttocks	tún	臀
MA-AH6	Sciatic Nerve	zuò gǔ shén jīng	坐骨神经
MA-AH7	Sympathetic	jiāo gǎn	交感
MA-AH	Lumbosacral Vertebrae	yāo dǐ zhuī	腰骶椎
MA-AH	Abdomen	fù	腹
MA-AH8	Cervical Vertebrae	jǐng zhuī	颈椎
MA-AH9	Thoracic Vertebrae	xiōng zhuī	胸椎
MA-AH10	Neck	jǐng	颈
MA-AH	Thyroid	jiǎ zhuàng xiàn	甲状腺
MA-AH11	Chest	xiōng	胸
MA-AH	Mammary Gland	rǔ xiàn	乳腺
MA-TF	Adnexa Uteri (ovary and fallopian tube)	fù jiàn	附件
MA-TF	Blood Pressure Lowering (Anterior)	jiàng yā diǎn	降压点
MA-TF	Superior Triangular Fossa	jiǎo wō shàng	角窝上
MA-TF	Internal Reproductive Organs	něi shēng zhí qì	内生殖器
MA-TF	Ovary	luǎn cháo	卵巢
MA-TF	Uterus	zǐ gōng	子宫
MA-TF	Cervix	gōng jǐn	宫颈
MA-TF	Middle Triangular Fossa	jiǎo wō zhōng	角窝中
MA-TF	Pelvis	pén qiāng	盆腔
MA-TF1	Ear Shén Mén	ěr shén mén	耳神门
MA-T	Adrenal Gland	shèn shàng xiàn	肾上腺
MA-T	Internal Nose	nèi bí	内鼻
MA-T	External Ear	wài ěr	外耳
MA-T	Upper Apex of Tragus	shàng píng jián	上屏尖
MA-T1	External Nose	wài bí	外鼻
MA-T2	Lower Apex of Tragus	xià píng jián	下屏尖
MA-T3	Pharynx and Larynx	yān hóu	咽喉

MA-AT	Apex of Antitragus	píng jiān	屏尖
MA-AT	Apex of Antitragus	duì píng jiān	对屏尖
MA-AT	Brain	năo diăn	脑点
MA-AT	Brain Stem	năo gàn	脑干
MA-AT	Calm Panting	píng chuăn	平喘
MA-AT	Central Rim	yuán zhōng	缘中
MA-AT	Forehead	é	额
MA-AT	Occiput	zhĕn	枕
MA-AT	Parotid	sāi xiàn	腮腺
MA-AT1	Subcortex	pí zhì xià	皮质下
MA-AT	Temple	niè	颞
MA-AT	Testicle	găo wán	睾丸
MA-AT	Vertigo	xuán yūn	眩晕
MA-IC	Heart	xīn	心
MA-IC	Spleen	pĭ	脾
MA-IC	Stomach	wèi	胃
MA-IC1	Lung	fèi	肺
MA-IC2	Bronchii/Trachea	qì guăn	气管
MA-IC3	Endocrine	nèi fēn mì	内分泌
MA-IC4	Triple Burner	sān jiāo	三焦
MA-IC5	Mouth	kŏu	口
MA-IC6	Esophagus	shí dào	食道
MA-IC7	Cardiac	pēn mén	贲门
MA-SC	Biliary Duct	dăn dào	胆道
MA-SC	Drunkenness	zuì diăn	醉点
MA-SC	Prostate [Angle of Superior Concha]	qián liè xiàn	前列腺
MA-SC	Angle of Superior Concha [Prostate]	tĭng jiāo	艇角
MA-SC	Kidney	shèn	肾
MA-SC	Middle of Superior Concha	tĭng zhōng	艇中
MA-SC1	Duodenum	shí èr zhĭ cháng	十二指肠
MA-SC2	Small Intestine	xiăo cháng	小肠
MA-SC3	Appendix	lán wĕi	阑尾
MA-SC4	Large Intestine	dà cháng	大肠
MA-SC5	Liver	gān	肝

MA-SC6	Pancreas/Gallbladder	yí dǎn	胰胆
MA-SC7	Ureter	shū niào guǎn	输尿管
MA-SC8	Bladder	páng guāng	膀胱
MA-L	Anterior Ear Lobe	chuí qián	垂前
MA-L	Eye 1	mù1	目 1
MA-L	Eye 2	mù2	目 2
MA-L	Internal Ear	něi ěr	内耳
MA-L	Cheek	miàn jiá	面颊
MA-L	Jaw	hé	颌
MA-L	Tongue	shé	舌
MA-L	Tonsil	biǎn táo tǐ	扁桃体
MA-L	Tooth	yá	牙
MA-L	Blood Pressure Raising (Anterior)	shēng yā diǎn	升压点
MA-L1	Eye	yǎn	眼
MA-PS	Lower Ear Root	xià ěr gēn	下耳根
MA-PS	Lung of Posterior Surface	ěr bèi fèi	耳背肺
MA-PS	Upper Ear Root	shàng ěr gēn	上耳根
MA-PS	Blood Pressure-Lowering Groove	jiàng yā gōu	降压沟
MA-PS	Blood Pressure-Raising Groove	shēng yā gōu	升压沟
MA-PS	Groove of Posterior Surface	ěr bèi gōu	耳背沟
MA-PS	Heart of Posterior Surface	ěr bèi xīn	耳背心
MA-PS	Kidney of Posterior Surface	ěr bèi shèn	耳背肾
MA-PS	Liver of Posterior Surface	ěr bèi gān	耳背肝
MA-PS	Root of Ear Vagus	ěr mí gēn	耳迷根
MA-PS	Spleen of Posterior Surface	ěr bèi pǐ	耳背脾

INDEX

Modern Chinese Ear Acupuncture Chart
Ping Chen, C.M.D, O.M.D.

This is an attractive, finely detailed, and graphically enhanced full color wall chart showing all the points, areas, and groupings on the anterior and posterior of the ear surface. Each of roughly 80 points and areas is identified with the English name, the international standard name reference, Pinyin name, and Chinese characters, and each is color-coded by its location. Both anterior and posterior anatomical areas are detailed. It conforms to the point location and treatment information to be found in *Modern Chinese Ear Acupuncture* by Ping Chen. This chart is certain to be received as the most complete and accurate chart reference for Chinese ear acupuncture available to date. (Measures 36" x 23".)

Ordering Information

Phone: 800-873-3946 or 505-758-7758

Fax 505-758-7768

Email: orders@redwingbooks.com

Website: www.redwingbooks.com